OSCEsmart

50 Medical Student OSCEs
in Emergency Medicine

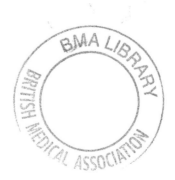

Dr. Dilhan Perusinghe

Executive Consulting Editor:
Dr. Sam Thenabadu

Ordering Information: Quantity sales. Special discounts are available on quantity purchases by corporations, associations, and others. For details, contact the publisher at the address above.

Orders by UK trade bookstores and wholesalers please visit www.scowenpublishing.com

Although every effort has been made to check this text, it is possible that errors have been made, readers are urged to check with the most up to date guidelines and safety regulations.

The authors and the publishers do not accept responsibility or legal liability for any errors in the text, or for the misuse of the material in this book.

Publisher's Cataloging-in-Publication data : OSCEsmart 50 medical student OSCEs in Emergency Medicine.

ISBN: 0-9908538-7-X

ISBN-13: 978-0-9908538-7-9

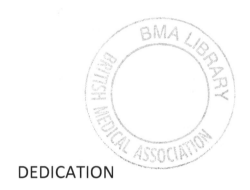

DEDICATION

'The world is full of great teachers. Having the opportunity to learn from them is fortuitous but having the opportunity to teach that knowledge is a blessing. Thanks to my brother who taught me growing up, and thanks to the greatest teacher of all, my Mother.'

Dilhan

'For Ammi, Molly, Reuben and Rafa - I.L.Y.T.T.M.'

Sam

CONTENTS

Message from the authors

Doctors of all seniorities can remember the stress of the OSCE but even more so the stress of trying to study and practice for the OSCEs. A multitude of generic undergraduate and postgraduate resources can be found on line but quality, quantity, and completeness of content can vary. The aim of the OSCESmart editorial team is to bring together specialty focused books that have identified 50 core stations encompassing the essential categories of history taking, examinations, emergency moulages, clinical skills and data interpretation with a strong theme of communications running through all the stations.

The combined experience of consultants, registrars and junior doctors to write, edit and quality check these stations, promises to deliver content that is appropriate to reach a standard we would expect of new junior doctors entering their foundation internship years and into core training. It is important to know that these stations are all newly written and based at the level of clinical competencies we would expect from these grades of doctors. Learning objectives exist for undergraduate curricula and for the foundation years, and the scenarios are based and written around these. What they are not, are scenarios that have been 'borrowed' from any medical school.

Preparation is the key to success in most things, but never more so than for the OSCEs and a candidate that hasn't practised will soon be found out. These books will allow you to practice relevant scenarios with verified checklists to learn both content and the generic approach. The format will allow you to practice in groups with one person being the candidate, one the actor and one the examiner. Each scenario finishes with three learning points. Picture these as are three core learning tips that we would want you to take away if you had only a couple of days left to the exam. These OSCE scenarios promise to be a robust revision aide for the student looking to recap and consolidate for their exams, but equally importantly prepare them for life in clinical practice.

I am immensely proud of this OSCESmart series. I have had the pleasure of working with some of the brightest and most dynamic young clinicians and educators I know, and I am sure you will find this series covering the essential clinical specialties a truly robust and invaluable companion in those stressful times of revision. I must take this opportunity to thank my colleagues for all their hard work but most of all to thank my wonderful wife Molly for her unerring love and support and my sons Reuben and Rafael for all the joy they bring me.

Despite the challenging times the health service finds itself in, being a doctor remains a huge privilege. We hope that this OSCESmart series goes some way to help you achieve the excellence you and your patients deserve.

Best of luck,
Dr Sam Thenabadu

Introduction to OSCE Smart in Emergency Medicine

Emergency medicine is a rapidly growing field of medicine and changing field of medicine. With the acceptance of this specialty and the versatility that it offers we now have more trainees than ever. University Colleges are recognising this and the importance of training students to deal with emergencies. Regardless of whichever specialty someone chooses, there will always be a need to learn how to deal with emergencies. The most effective way to remember how to treat emergencies and to keep a cool head is to have practiced these thought processes and actions repeatedly. Practicing them so much that they become second nature and no longer require thinking.

OSCE's are the one place where star candidates can fall down. Nerves can better us in any high-pressure situation but particularly in emergency scenarios. We can eliminate nerves through rehearsal of these scenarios. 50 Smart Osces in EM teaches a structured approach that will not only help pass your exams but will also help in those moments that count with sick patients in the hospital.

During this book we take the student through a mixture of realistic scenarios. We begin with A-E assessments - the key to assessing sick patients quickly, systematically and safely. 80% of a diagnosis comes from a history. The next section allows you to practice the succinct history taking stations from exams. This is an opportunity to mastering the words you use when speaking to a formal patient. The next section allows us to practice our examinations. Choice examinations have been picked that are guaranteed to be tested repeatedly from med' school through to specialty training.

The next set of stations are practical skills. Familiarising yourself with these will ensure that you look comfortable and natural when performing in the OSCE. These are ideal to perform in the clinical skills room at your Uni or hospital. The final stop in this OSCE journey is data interpretation a skill you will use daily but is very rarely taught and practiced. Substituting various ABG's, ECGs or CXR's.

Practicing for your osces can be a fun! Our scenarios are designed so that like minded friends can get together and learn how each role perceives the candidate. Clear instructions for your friends (medical or non-medical) are given in each scenario so that everyone can play the different roles easily as well as enjoy some Oscar grade acting.

I would like to give a special thanks to the Co-authors of this book and of course Dr Sam Thenabadu whose passion for education continues to inspire both myself and my colleagues. Good luck studying!

Dilhan Perusinghe

About the Authors

Dr Dilhan Perusinghe

MBBS MEng
CT3 Emergency Medicine

Having started his higher education in Medical Engineering, Dr Perusinghe found himself changing his focus from numbers, to people, from a world of building, design and machines, to a lifetime dedicated to one marvelous machine.

He first worked in a busy emergency department at a trauma centre in the University Hospital Coventry and Warwickshire (UHCW). After working in this team full of efficient, fun and sometimes crazy people, he knew there was no possibility of return to the mundane.

Every case was an opportunity to learn and a number of great teachers schooled him through his learning. He worked a further year as an Emergency Medicine clinical fellow at UHCW. Arriving in London for his training, he spent time with Dr Thenabadu at the Princess Royal University Hospital. Here he started learning more about the art of teaching, as well as honing his own knowledge and skill set.

He progressed through his ACCS training and is currently working in his ST3 year as a Paediatric Emergency Department doctor in University Hospital Lewisham.

Dr Sam Thenabadu

MBBS MRCP DRCOG DCH MA Clin Ed FRCEM MSc (Paed) FHEA

Consultant Adult & Paediatric Emergency Medicine
Honorary Senior Lecturer & Associate Director of Medical Education

Sam Thenabadu graduated from King's College Medical School in 2001 and dual trained in Adult and Paediatric Emergency Medicine in London before being appointed a consultant in 2011 at the Princess Royal University Hospital. He has Masters degrees in Clinical Medical Education and Advanced Paediatrics.

He is undergraduate director of medical education at the King's College NHS Trust and the academic block lead for Emergency Medicine and Critical Care at King's College School of Medicine. At postgraduate level he has been the Pan London Health Education England lead for CT3 paediatric emergency medicine trainees since 2011. Academically he has previously written two textbooks and has published in peer review journals and given numerous oral and poster presentations at national conferences in emergency medicine, paediatrics, medical education and patient quality and safety.

He has an unashamed passion for medical education and strives to achieve excellence for himself, his colleagues and his patients, hoping to always deliver this through an enjoyable learning environment. Service delivery and educational need not be two separate entities, and he hopes that those who have had great teachers will take it upon themselves to do the same for others in the future.

Co Authors

Dr Amy Attwater MBChB (Hons) BSc (Hons)
Staff Grade Clinical fellow in Emergency Medicine, University
Hospital Coventry and Warwickshire

Dr Thomas Peter Fox MBBS MRCEM
ST3 Emergency Medicine, University Hospital Lewisham, London

Dr Yannic N.P. Graichen, BMBS, BMedSci,
ST3 Emergency medicine, Guy's and St Thomas' Hospital, London

Dr Atul Kapoor
ST3 Emergency Medicine, Guy's and St Thomas' Hospital, London

Dr Claire Kilbride MBChB
CT2 Emergency Medicine, Guy's and St Thomas' Hospital, London

Dr Marthani Maheswaran MBBS BSc MRCEM
ST3 Emergency Medicine Homerton University Hospital

Dr Alexander C E Robertson, MBChB BSc MRCEM
ST3 Emergency Medicine, The Royal London Hospital

Dr Siobhan Roche, MBChB
CT2 Emergency medicine, Guy's and St Thomas' Hospital, London

Dr Sarah Schneider, MBChB, BMedSci Hons,
CT1 Emergency Medicine trainee, Princess Royal University
Hospital

Dr Amy Servante, Bsc(Hons) MBBS
ST3 Emergency Medicine, King's College Hospital, London

Abbreviations

AAA – Abdominal aorta aneurysm
ABCDE – Airway, Breathing, Circulation, Disability, Exposure
ATLS – Advance Trauma Life Support
BD – Twice a day
BPH - Benign Prostatic Hyperplasia
BPM – Beats Per Minute
C-Spine – Cervical Spine
CT - Computerised tomography
CT IVU - Computerised tomography intravenous urogram
CXR – Chest Radiograph
DNAR - Do Not Attempt Resuscitation
DRE – Digital Rectal Examination
ERCP - Endoscopic Retrograde cholangiopancreatography
FNA- Fine Needle Aspiration
GORD - Gastro-oesophageal reflux disease
GP - General practitioner
ITU – Intensive Care Unit
IHD – Ischemic Heart Disease
MRCP - Magnetic resonance cholangiopancreatography
RUQ- Right upper quadrant
OD – Once a day
OSCEs - objective structured clinical examinations
PCA – Pain Control Analgesia
PRN- As when Required
PSA – Prostate-specific antigen
P-POSSUM – risk calculation in a preoperative patient
SOCRATES - mnemonic acronym used evaluate the nature of pain
TIA- Transient Ischemic Attack
USS - Ultrasound

Chapter One

A to E Moulage Scenarios

1. Splenic Injury

Candidate's instructions

You are the Foundation doctor in the ED and you have been asked by the trauma team leader to perform a primary survey.

A 31-year-old cyclist is brought into the Emergency Department resuscitation room having had a collision with a van going at 30MPH. Currently the patient is fully conscious, Glasgow Coma Score (GCS) 15. Their pulse is 110 beats per minute and their blood pressure is 90/50mmHg. He has been moved to the resuscitation room and has a C-spine collar in place. The trauma team are present.

Please perform the primary survey examination, present the relevant findings to the team and suggest a management plan.

Examiner's instructions

A 31 year-old cyclist has been brought into the emergency department resuscitation room as part of a trauma call. The candidate has been asked to perform the primary survey on the patient, take a focused history and to relate their findings back to the trauma team leader.

At 6 minutes, or before if the candidate has finished, you should ask the candidate to summarise their findings and suggest a management plan.

The candidate should give a succinct summary of the findings of the primary survey. The candidate should highlight the likely diagnosis of an injury to the spleen and major blood loss.

A- The airway is patent and the patient is allowed to respond to questioning so that we can prove it is patent.

B - Their oxygen saturation are 99% on room air however a non-rebreathe mask should be placed in as this is a trauma.

C- They have a low blood pressure 90/50 and have a high pulse rate 110bpm. They will have pain in their left upper abdomen, this is consistent with an injury to the spleen and major blood loss.

D- GCS 15 and BM 5.1

E - If the candidate asks to fully expose the patient, inform them that in this scenario the patient has been fully exposed and no external injury was found.

Actor's instruction

Patient: you will respond to simple questions from the candidate about your name, age and date of birth and current location. You have been in an accident. You were cycling when a van travelling the opposite direction veered into you. You hit the windscreen and landed behind the van. You did not lose consciousness. You were wearing a helmet. You have a few cuts and scrapes. The only pain you have is in your abdomen. When the candidate examines your abdomen you will respond as if it is sore when they feel the upper left hand side. You will be wearing a neck brace and will have a block on either side of your head, taped to the mattress. (For comfort you can tell the candidate that this is in place)

If the candidate asks for a "log roll" you will be rolled onto your side by the other actors in the team and the candidate will press on your spine from head to lower back. You will respond that you can feel the candidate touching your back and that it is not painful.

Trauma team members

Anaesthetist: You will stay at the head end of the patient, confirm there is no airway problem and lead the log roll if the candidate requests to do one.

Resus Nurse 1: You will perform the vital sign observations; respiratory rate is 16, oxygen saturation 99% on room air, the blood pressure is 90/50mmHg, and pulse 110bpm. You will inform the candidate that the patient has intravenous access when asked. His haemoglobin will be 70 on the venous gas and the rest of the blood tests will be pending.

Mark Scheme

Task:	Achieved	Not Achieved
Washes hands and Introduces self to patient		
Clarifies who the team are and their role		
Elicits a brief history		
Comments that Airway is Clear/Confirms C spine protection		
Asks for oxygen saturation and respiratory rate		
Auscultates chest wall and comments good air entry on both sides		
Palpates chest wall and comments no pain response, good chest wall expansion		
Asks for BP and feels for pulse		
Requests large bore cannulation bloods including FBC, Group and Screen		
Recognises haemorrhage due to hypotension and tachycardia, suggests calling a code red (major haemorrhage protocol) and fluid resuscitation		
Examines abdomen elicits tenderness in left upper quadrant		
Palpates pelvis		
Asks for patient to be fully exposed		
Asks for blood sugar level		
Asks for a Log roll and correctly examines the back		
Ascertains GCS		
Presents summary of A to E assessment		
Gives and appropriate differential diagnosis including splenic laceration		
Suggests appropriate management plan		
Explains needs to go to theatre for a laparotomy		
Examiners Global Mark	/5	
Actor/Helpers Global Mark	/5	
Total Station Mark	/30	

4

Learning Points

- A well-rehearsed and systematic primary survey is essential to not miss any injury in a trauma patient. Using the A to E template ensures that all team members are aware of the structure and that findings aren't missed.

- Haemodynamic instability in a trauma patient with abdominal pain needs to be treated as a major haemorrhage with appropriate fluid resuscitation however the definitive management is a laparotomy. A major haemorrhage protocol may need to be declared and tranexamic acid can be given to help manage bleeding.

- Communication is a key factor in treating the trauma patient. The trauma team leader relies on succinct reports from all members of the team to organise the appropriate investigation and management of a trauma patient.

2. Long bone fracture

Candidate's instructions

You are the foundation doctor in the ED working in the resuscitation area. You are alerted to a trauma call, which is due to arrive imminently.

A 62-year-old man has been injured following a collision with a car. The patient is GCS 15, HR 120, BP 120/80, has a deformed left leg and is requiring morphine for pain control. No other injuries have been noted.

Your registrar is busy and has asked you to take handover from the paramedics and perform a primary survey, taking steps to address any bleeding and pain. You have another foundation doctor and a senior nurse to help you. A cubicle in the resuscitation area has been fully prepared, you have one minute before the patient's arrival to organise your team.

Actor's instructions

You are a 62-year-old architect who was hit by a car this morning. You have been given some morphine but are still in pain and very anxious.

You are not able to provide the doctor with any further information due to pain and anxiety. You are fully alert and keep asking for something to take the pain away.

Paramedic handover

This is a 62-year-old patient who was involved in a road traffic collision about 50 minutes ago.

He was hit on the left side by a vehicle turning a corner at about 25 miles per hour. His leg gave way immediately and he fell to the floor. Witnesses state he was not thrown into the air and he did not hit the windscreen or go under the vehicle.

He has a deformity to the left leg but no other notable injuries. He strongly denies any head, neck or back pain. Witnesses state he did not lose consciousness and he was conversing normally when the paramedics arrived on scene.

He has a history of a myocardial infarction and takes bisoprolol and aspirin. He states he is not allergic to anything and last ate at 8am.

His initial BP was 120/80, HR 120, Sats 100% on air. Both feet were pink and he can move his toes. We have inserted a cannula and administered a total of 10mg IV morphine.

Examiner's Instructions

The foundation doctor has been asked to see a 62-year-old patient who has sustained a closed mid-shaft femoral fracture following a collision with a car. There has been a significant haemorrhage from the fracture site (consistent with a class II haemorrhage). They have no other injuries.

The candidate has been asked to take handover from the paramedics, perform a primary survey and implement any immediate resuscitation and management, with a focus on haemorrhage control and analgesia. The patient has no cervical spine immobilisation on arrival, despite the paramedics insisting, but he hasn't complained of neck pain. A hard collar, straps and blocks should be placed due to the presence of a distracting injury. The other doctor can fit this.

The candidate should take steps to address the bleeding source by realigning and immobilising the fractured limb (a Thomas splint is available). The other doctor cannot apply a splint. If the candidate asks for a trauma call to be placed, an orthopaedic surgeon will arrive one minute before the end of the scenario and the rest of the team are on their way.

As the patient is examined and monitoring is placed the following is found:

Appearance - In pain and anxious.

A & C-Spine - Patent. Talking. Neck is not immobilised.

B - Normal appearance of the chest. Respiratory rate 22. Normal breathing pattern. Trachea is central. Normal palpation and percussion. Bilateral air entry. Sats 100% on 2 litres oxygen via nasal cannula.

C - Warm and well perfused. Capillary refill time 2 seconds. Pulse 90 regular. BP 130/80. Normal heart sounds. One 18 gauge peripheral venous access in situ. Pulses in the feet and ankles preserved but weak in the left (CRT 3 seconds in left foot).

D - GCS 15/15. Unable to move his left lower limb due to pain. Can wiggle toes bilaterally and sensation is preserved. Pupils size 3mm bilaterally and reactive. Blood glucose 7.6

E - Notably deformed, shortened and swollen left thigh with extensive skin discolouration (deep red-purple), no laceration to skin, no visible bone. Mild soft tissue damage over the right thigh. No other notable injury. Abdomen is soft and non-tender. Temperature 36ºC

Mark Scheme

Task	Achieved	Not Achieved
Introduces themselves to the team and establishes experience		
Requests that a trauma call be placed		
Allocates roles/jobs to team members		
Washes hands and dons personal protective equipment and ensures that team members are protected		
Takes handover from the paramedics and promotes an appropriate environment		
Requests monitoring		
Immobilises the cervical spine		
Establishes airway is patient and not compromised		
Examines the chest. Notes raised respiratory rate		
Examines circulation. Notes they are tachycardic		
Obtains further IV access and starts fluid or blood resuscitation.		
Notes GCS/AVPU and examines pupils.		
Fully exposes. Identifies injuries. Checks temperature and keeps warm.		
Identifies the need to realign and immobilise the leg		
Checks neurovascular status of the limb before splint is applied		
Provides further analgesia		
Applies a Thomas splint correctly		
Checks neurovascular status of the limb after splint is applied		
Hands over to the orthopaedic surgeon appropriately		
Communicates well with the team throughout		
Examiner's Global Mark	/5	
Actor / Helper's Global Mark	/5	
Total Station Mark	/30	

Learning points

- One of the main skills of the trauma team leader is to provide clear structure and direction to a potentially chaotic situation. When being examined on these scenarios it is likely that you are being scored on your communication, team working and leadership skills as well as clinical knowledge.

- A traction splint aims to realign the limb and give an element of stability, thus reducing pain and minimising the risk of neurological and vascular complications. Realigning a fractured limb can reduce the bleeding from the fracture site and it therefore forms part of your circulation assessment.

- Cervical spine immobilisation is a heavily debated topic in emergency medicine but is fairly straightforward when it comes to an OSCE - if in a trauma scenario you are expected to immobilise the cervical spine. Be familiar with the NICE, Canadian and NEXUS clinical rules for cervical spine immobilisation and clearance.

3. Tension Pneumothorax

Candidate's Instructions

You are a foundation doctor working in the Emergency Department of a district general hospital. An ambulance is on its way with a 27-year-old male cyclist who was hit by a car. His C-spine has been immobilised by the ambulance team.

Please assess this patient, stating any interventions you would like to perform as you go along.

Examiner's Instructions

A 27-year-old male cyclist who was hit by a car is being brought to the Emergency Department by ambulance. His C-spine has been triple immobilised by the ambulance team.

If asked by the candidate, please provide the following information:
The trauma team are on their way to assist you but you must start your assessment immediately.

A – Patent, no obvious facial deformities, no upper airway noises

B – RR 42, oxygen saturations are 74% on room air, 86% on high flow oxygen, significantly increased work of breathing, right side of chest not moving with respiration, decreased air entry to right side of chest on auscultation, right side of chest hyper-resonant on percussion and mild tracheal deviation.

C – Pulse rate 120, blood pressure 88/50, cool peripheries, sweaty, capillary refill time 3 seconds

D – GCS 14/15, confused and agitated

E – Few superficial cuts and bruises to the lower limbs, no limb deformities.
Once candidate states/performs needle decompression, saturations improve to 99%, HR decreases to 90 and BP starts to improves to 110/80. Ask what the candidates next management would be ideally this would be to speak to ITU and to start the insertion of a chest drain.

Actor's Instructions:

You are a staff nurse in the Emergency Department. You are able to assist the candidate and you know where all the equipment is kept. You are not able to perform tasks unless clearly instructed to by the candidate.

Mark Scheme

Task	Achieved	Not Achieved
Appropriate introduction and task allocation to team members		
Calls early for trauma team		
Ensures all members of the team wear appropriate PPE		
Ensures C-spine immobilisation throughout assessment		
Appropriate assessment of patient's airway		
Assessment of breathing - RR, oxygen saturations, work of breathing, auscultation, percussion		
Administers oxygen via appropriate device		
Assessment of circulation - BP, HR, capillary refill time		
States would like to gain IV/IO access and send appropriate samples to laboratory		
States would like to commence IV/IO fluids		
Assessment of neurological status		
Adequately exposes patient to look for other injuries or bruising		
Makes diagnosis of tension pneumothorax		
States would like to perform immediate needle decompression		
States correct anatomical landmarks for procedure (2nd ICS MCL)		
Reassesses patient after intervention has been made		
States definitive management is a chest drain		
Correctly identifies landmarks for insertion of chest drain		
Considers need for imaging (CXR)		
Demonstrates systematic A-E assessment		
Examiner's Global Mark	/5	
Actor / Helper's Global Mark	/5	
Total Station Mark	/30	

Learning points

- Tension pneumothorax is a clinical diagnosis, which needs immediate management with needle decompression. This is performed by inserting a large-bore cannula in the 2nd intercostal space, in the mid-clavicular line on the affected side. This relieves the tension and converts the injury to a simple pneumothorax, which will subsequently need definitive treatment with insertion of a chest drain.

- In a trauma scenario, it is important to have a systematic process to assessing patients. The A (and C-spine) BCDE technique is easy to remember and ensures that you do not miss any injuries. Remember to treat life-threatening injuries as you go along and reassess the patient after you have made an intervention. If there is a B problem then make an intervention before you move on.

- In order to assess breathing and ventilation, adequately expose the patient's chest and use all information available to you, including inspection for any open injuries, bruising of the chest wall, work of breathing and movement of the chest. Oxygen saturations and respiratory rate provide valuable information as does thorough auscultation and percussion of the chest.

4. ALS: PEA arrest

Candidate's Instructions:

You are a foundation doctor working in the Emergency Department when you discover a 60-year-old unresponsive male in a cubicle. Assess and manage this patient according to the principles of Advanced Life Support.

After 6 minutes the examiner will stop you and ask you to summarise back your findings and your management plan.

Examiner's Instructions:

A 60-year-old male has become unresponsive in a cubicle in the emergency department. The doctor has discovered this patient and is willing to lead the resuscitation.

The candidate must do this according to the principles of ALS.

After 6 minutes stop the candidate whatever stage they are at and ask them to 'please summarise your findings and your management plan from here'

Actor's Instructions:

A manikin will usually be used for this scenario.

Mark Scheme: ALS PEA

Task	Achieved	Not Achieved
Checks it is safe to approach		
Establishes patient unresponsive, not breathing and pulseless (look,listen and feel for 10s)		
Calls for help/activates emergency buzzer		
Commences CPR (at correct position and depth)		
Attached defibrillator pads when help arrives/delegated		
Correctly assesses rhythm as PEA		
Asks for pulse check (3 point check)		
Continues chest compressions immediately - 100-120/min		
Switches to 30:2 now help has arrived w BVM		
Establishes intravenous access		
Gives 1mg of Adrenaline IV (1:10000)as soon as possible		
Secure the airway – iGel or intubation		
Switches from 30:2 to continuous CPR once airway secured		
Rhythm and pulse check after 2 minutes		
Continues CPR		
Ensures high quality of chest compressions (1/3rd of chest depth)		
Gives 1mg Adrenaline IV every 3-5 minutes		
Mentions reversible causes of cardiac arrest (4H's, 4T's)		
Identifies return of pulse		
Commences post resuscitation care		
Examiner's Global Mark	/5	
Actor / Helper's Global Mark	/5	
Total Station Mark	/30	

Learning Points

- Be well versed with the ALS algorithm for shockable (VT/VF) and non-shockable (PEA/asystole) rhythms.

- Have a good grasp of the reversible causes of cardiac arrest and their management:

  Hypoxia
  Hypovolaemia
  Hyperkalaemia, hypokalaemia, hypoglycaemia,
  hypocalcaemia, acidaemia and other metabolic disorders
  Hypothermia

  Thrombosis (coronary or pulmonary)
  Tension pneumothorax
  Tamponade – cardiac
  Toxins

- If a diagnosis of asystole is made, check the ECG carefully for the presence of P waves. The patient may respond to cardiac pacing when there is ventricular standstill with continuing P waves. There is no value in attempting to pace true asystole.

5. ALS: VF arrest

Candidate's instructions

You are the foundation doctor on call for general medicine. The crash bleep goes off and tells you that there is an arrest on the ward next to yours. You are the first of the crash team to arrive on the ward.

Helper's instructions:

You are a newly qualified nurse on the general medical ward. Mr Jones was admitted today with chest pain. He was awaiting a repeat troponin (cardiac blood test) and had been given ACS treatment in the meantime.

He had a heart attack about 3 years ago and you are unaware of any other past medical history.

5 minutes ago he had developed central crushing chest pain then became unresponsive with no pulse or respiratory effort. You started chest compressions and called for a colleague to put out a cardiac arrest call.

When the doctor arrives you are anxious but are able to hand over all of the information above. Your college has brought the defibrillator however they are unable to stay.

From here on you follow the instructions given by the candidate.

Examiner's instructions:

This station examines the candidate's knowledge of the ALS protocol. When the candidate arrives on scene the nurse has already started performing chest compressions. They should confirm the cardiac arrest themselves.

They will need prompting with examination findings should they ask for them throughout the scenario.

When the pads are attached pause for a rhythm and pulse check. The monitor will show a VF arrest. They should identify this as a 'shockable rhythm' and instruct for CPR to be resumed.

Once they have delivered one shock and asked for CPR to be restarted, ask the candidate to tell you how long they would continue compressions for before they check the rhythm (answer 2 minutes)?

Once this has been covered tell them that their 2 minutes are up. They should recheck the rhythm. The patient has returned to normal sinus rhythm and the candidate should check the pulse to confirm that this is not PEA.

You can then end the scenario and ask the following questions:

1. Which drugs are used in a VF arrest situation and when are they given?

    Adrenaline and Amiodarone are given after the third shock only in a VF arrest.

2. Can you list the 8 reversible causes of cardiac arrest?

    (4 H's) - Hypoxia, Hypothermia, Hypo/hyperkalaemia and other electrolyte abnormalities and Hypovolaemia, (4 T's) – Tamponade, Tension pneumothorax, Thrombus and Toxins

Extra marks are awarded for good communication with their team.

Mark Scheme: VF Arrest

Task	Achieved	Not Achieved
Introduces self to nurse on scene		
Confirms cardiac arrest		
Puts on defibrillating pads and pauses for rhythm check		
Identifies VF on monitor		
Identifies VF as a shockable rhythm		
Communicates the need for a shock to be delivered		
Requests chest compressions to be restarted immediately after rhythm has been identified		
Reassures compression nurse that she will not be shocked		
Selects a setting of at least 150J and charges the defibrillator		
Requests that everyone stand clear		
Requests that oxygen is kept clear		
Briefly checks that everyone is clear of the patient and safely delivers shock		
Requests for chest compressions to be started immediately after delivery of shock		
Knows that CPR should be continued for another 2 minutes after shock		
Inserts IV access or suggests alternative access		
Correctly identifies normal sinus rhythm and checks for pulse		
Communicates well with members of the team		
Knows that adrenaline should be administered after the third shock and every 3-5 minutes thereafter		
Knows that amiodarone 300mg should be administered after the third shock		
Correctly lists 4H's and 4T's		
Examiner's Global Mark	/5	
Actor / Helper's Global Mark	/5	
Total Station Mark	/30	

Learning points

- As the clinician running the arrest the temptation is to get drawn in. Stand back, observe and delegate to the rest of the team. A team will function far better with an allocated leader to coordinate the multiple interventions that are ongoing. In addition to the leader, roles are needed for managing the airway, the defibrillator, performing chest compressions, delivering drugs and scribing.

- Communication is imperative in this situation. It is very useful to use closed-loop communication. This means that you give an instruction to one person specifically and ask them to give you feedback when they have carried it out. This ensures that you are well informed about what your team members are doing.

- Ask a competent assistant to manage the airway as much are they are able to. Early use of the supra-glottic airway allows for continuous compression and ventilation to take place. Once the airway is secure check for good bilateral air entry.

For the full ALS algorithm see www.resus.org.uk

6. Anaphylaxis

Candidate's Instructions

You are the foundation doctor in the Emergency Department in the resus area overnight. A 19-year-old man gets brought in by ambulance after being picked up outside a kebab shop where they have reported difficulty in breathing. They have also been noted to have developed a widespread rash and prominent lip swelling.

The ambulance crew hand over that they don't think there is any Past medical history.

Please assess and manage this patient.

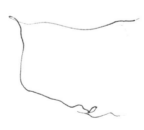

Examiner's Instructions

This 19-year-old gets brought into ED resus at 2am. They've been brought in by ambulance after being picked up outside a kebab shop where the patient said they suddenly could not breathe and was noted to have developed a rash with lip swelling.

The foundation doctor in resus overnight has been asked to assess and manage this patient.

They should follow a methodical A to E approach:

A - The girl will become increasingly short of breath and wheezy if oxygen isn't given as part of A. Lip swelling noted (Angioedema).

The candidate should also know that even though medicines usually come later in an A-E assessment, 500mcg 1:1000 adrenaline IM and 10mg chlorphenamine IV(or other antihistamine of choice) should be given in the first instance of anaphylaxis during assessment.

If the candidate asks for an anaesthetist/ICU to be bleeped, they will be enroute ASAP, but are currently delayed in theatre.

B - The patient will struggle to talk or breathe given her SOB, wheeziness and lip swelling. O2 saturations read 92-94%. Reduced air entry at lung bases but loud upper airway sounds on auscultation with inspiratory stridor. Salbutamol and Ipratropium bromide can be given at this point.

Candidate will have difficulties eliciting a history from her till later in the assessment when she's had treatment.

C - IV fluids will need to be given through 2 large bore cannulae. Bloods can be taken at this point. ABG is also appropriate

D - GCS 15 and Glucose is 5 (normal)

E - Widespread, itchy, blanching rash on chest, arms and legs.

Continually re-assess ABCDE again post intervention.

2nd stage of re-assessing:

O2 has come up to 100%. BP has dropped to 80/50.

Part two for examiner to read out:

"The nurse notifies you that the patient has fallen asleep and she sounds like she's snoring."

3rd stage of re-assessing:

Reassess again from A-E and fast bleep anaesthetists:

After 5 minutes if there is an ongoing reaction more adrenaline can be given 500mcg of 1:1000 IM or only if expert seniors are present 50mcg of 1:10000 IV

They need to attempt airway maneuvers and insert an airway adjunct. Shows how to size and insert Guedel airway appropriately.

Only after they've done airway maneuvers with an airway adjunct do the anesthetists arrive.

Actor's Instructions

You are a 19-year-old man who has anaphylactic reactions to peanuts. You have forgotten your epipen on this evening out and didn't think you would need it. You have eaten a kebab, which has been cooked in peanut oil and immediately have started struggling to breathe with lip swelling and a widespread rash. You can't speak apart from pant and wheeze loudly.

By the 2nd round of re-assessment you are starting to feel a bit better and still panting but can say 4 word sentences. However, you feel your heart is racing and can't stop shaking.

By the 3rd stage of re-assessment, you fall asleep and start snoring and wheezing loudly.

Mark Scheme: Anaphylaxis

Task	Achieved	Not Achieved
Introduces self		
Call for help/bleep anaesthetists/senior review		
Assess patency of airway (speaking/GCS/additional sounds)		
OXYGEN 100% given immediately		
Asks for respiratory rate & pulse oximetry		
Chest auscultation for wheeze		
Salbutamol and ipratropium bromide nebs given		
Can consider an ABG and/or portable CXR		
GIVE ADRENALINE 500mcg of 1:1000 IM adrenaline (can be given earlier than this point)		
Lie flat and raise legs		
Checks BP, HR & CRT		
IV crystalloid fluid challenge through 2 wide bore cannulae		
Bloods to be sent off e.g. Mast cell tryptase		
Chlorphenamine 10mg IV		
Hydrocortisone 200mg IV		
GCS examination and glucose		
Expose patient looking for rashes		
Reassess patient after each intervention		
recognise need for airway manoeuvres or airway adjuncts (Correctly size and insert airway adjunct)		
Ask for anaesthetic review required urgently and considers 2nd dose of Adrenaline after 5 minutes		
Examiner's Global Mark	/5	
Actor / Helper's Global Mark	/5	
Total Station Mark	/30	

Learning Points

- Practice, practice, practice! The A-E approach should become second nature to you so that every patient you approach (real or simulated), should be managed in the acute setting in the same way. It will ensure safe practice and good methods of managing and resuscitating unwell patients.

- In moulage scenarios, expect the patient to go off! If they do, remember to remain calm and re-assess again. Anaphylaxis is a good example of where interventions need reassessment but that scenarios can deteriorate even despite treatments. Going back to A in the A-E approach will ensure that nothing is missed.

- Adrenaline in this scenario should be given as soon as anaphylaxis is recognized regardless of which stage of the A-E assessment you are on. Imtramuscular adrenaline is the first line route and if a patient has their own adrenaline auto injector with them (eg Epipen, Jext) it is fine to use this in the first instance.

7. Asthma

Candidate's Instructions

You are a foundation doctor in the Emergency Department who has been asked to see this 35-year-old asthmatic who has been brought around by the triage nurse. The nurse informs you he is an office worker who had just walked in and was found to have oxygen saturations of 93% and is struggling to complete sentences.

Please take a short history and examine the patient. Start treatment as appropriate.

Actor's Instructions

You are a 35-year-old salesman who is just back at work after a weekend away in the country. You noticed a bit of chest tightness and wheeze since the start of the weekend at the hotel and have had to use your inhalers more frequently. You have been taking the blue inhaler every couple of hours since last night and ran out of it at work. You also forgot to take the purple inhaler that you normally do each morning because you left it at the hotel.

You have had asthma since adolescence but it has been quite well controlled. The wheeze developed in your teens and you were prescribed a blue inhaler to help. You were started on a long acting purple inhaler the following year after your wheeze re-emerged. Your peak flow was last checked over 10 years ago and it was roughly 550 at best.

In the past 10 years you have only had to have nebulisers and steroids once in the hospital and did not stay the night. Your asthma is otherwise well controlled and you are compliant with medications using the **purple one daily** and **blue before exercise**.

You are supposed to be moderately breathless during the scenario, but doing this is quite difficult so it is important to try and say no more than 4 or 5 words before you take an extra breath or pause.

Examiner's Instructions

The candidate should take a short history and get an idea of severity of asthma attack. The patient has acute severe asthma with a PEFR of 220. He will benefit from nebulised salbutamol and ipratropium bromide as well as steroids in an appropriate dose. The candidate should select oxygen to drive the nebuliser. He can offer intravenous magnesium sulphate. He can ask for help from others for the therapies to be administered as well as help putting in an IV cannula or getting an arterial blood gas (ABG). The candidate should have an idea of features of life threatening asthma and a low threshold to ask for senior help.

As part of the assessment, you can provide the following information if asked.

A - patent
B - Trachea central,
Wheezy chest sounds, equal air entry, symmetrical chest rise, resonant to percussion
Observations: RR 28, SpO2 93%, PEFR 220. ABG PH 7.4 PO2 8.5 PCO2 4.1 HCO3 28
C - BP 120/70, HR 115, Cool peripheries
D - GCS 15/15
E - Afebrile, some cyanosis

After initial therapy

A - patent
B - Trachea central, clear breath sounds

Observations: RR 22, SpO2 99%, PEFR 450. ABG PH 7.4 PO2 13.5 PCO2 4.0 HCO3 28

C - BP 120/70, HR 120, cool peripheries
D - GCS 15/15
E - Afebrile

Mark Scheme

Task	Achieved	Not Achieved
Introduction and consent		
Takes appropriate history of presenting complaint		
Asks about medication and admission history		
Past medical history including atopy and smoking history		
Uses ABCDE approach		
Calls for help/ Provides O2		
Assess airway and trachea		
Assess breathing and ask for peak flow (ABG can be provided)		
Interprets peak flow chart		
Start nebuliser and steroid therapy		
Assess circulation and ask for IV cannula		
Assess disability (GCS and pupils) and exposure		
Reassess after initial treatment		
Knowledge of classifying severity of asthma attack		
Knowledge of admission criteria for asthma attack		
Knowledge of discharge criteria following asthma attack		
Aware of treatment ladder for asthma attack		
Criteria for chest xray/use of antibiotics/ ICU referral		
Early escalation for senior help		
An idea of appropriate follow up for asthma patients		
Examiner's Global Mark	/5	
Actor / Helper's Global Mark	/5	
Total Station Mark	/30	

Learning Points

- The peak expiratory flow rate is useful to determine severity of asthma. It is expressed as a percentage of the patients' previous best. If this is unavailable, then one can refer to the predicted PEFR chart for the patient's age and height. After treatment is administered the PEFR can be rechecked to see if there has been any improvement.

- Pulse oximetry determines the need for an arterial blood gas. Use supplemental oxygen to aim saturations between 94- 98%. If the saturations drop below 92% an arterial sample should be obtained for analysis.

- Blood gas analysis is useful as it can help diagnose the presence of life threatening asthma. This is when the PO2 is below 8kPa (very low) or the CO2 is normal (between 4.6 -6.0 kPa)

8. Bowel obstruction

Candidate's Instructions

You are the foundation doctor in the Emergency Department resus area awaiting an ambulance. On arrival the paramedics hand over that he is a 60-year-old man who has been vomiting every 1-2 hours for 2 days. The vomit was initially food coloured but is now brown and smelling offensive. He has not opened his bowels in 3 days. His wife tells the ambulance crew that he was referred to a specialist for a swelling in his right groin 2 months ago. Please assess the patient and treat as appropriate.

Examiner's Instructions

Provide the following information if requested:

A – Patent, patient is moaning but maintaining airway, no change on reassessment

B – RR 28, Sats 93% on air 98% with 15 L oxygen, normal air entry, no change on reassessment

C – HR 124, BP 85/43, capillary refill 3 seconds, peripherally vasoconstricted.

On re-assessment if IV fluids given. HR 100, BP 110/76, capillary refill time 2 seconds, no other changes.

D – GCS 10: eyes open to voice (3), Verbal – incomprehensible sounds (2), Localises to pain (5), moving all four limbs equally, does not change on reassessment

E – Hard tender swelling in right inguinal region not reducible, abdomen is generally distended, tender with high pitched bowel sounds, PR exam (not necessary to perform on actor)- empty rectum, no masses. Does not change on reassessment.

At an appropriate time ask the candidate to give their diagnosis, management plan, and who will they refer to?

Show the abdominal x-ray and ask them to describe it.

Actor's Instructions

You are a 60-year-old man with 2 days of frequent vomiting. You have not opened your bowels nor passed wind for 3 days. You noticed a swelling in your right groin 2 months ago, which has become harder and more painful for the past week. Your wife is concerned and calls an ambulance today.

If the candidate introduces themselves, or asks you for a response, you moan as if in pain, putting your hands on your abdomen, and open your eyes.

Your abdomen will be generally tender with some increased and localised tenderness in the right iliac fossa.

Mark Scheme: Bowel Obstruction

Task	Achieved	Not Achieved
Introduces self and washes hands		
Uses ABCDE approach		
Calls for help early senior ED/anaesthetics		
Checks airway patency		
Assesses breathing		
Gives oxygen appropriately		
Assesses circulation		
Recognises need for IV access/IV fluids		
Assesses GCS/gross neurology (disability)		
Exposes patient for examination and examines abdomen		
Mentions PR exam		
Reassesses ABCDE after patient vomiting		
Diagnoses likely bowel obstruction		
Management includes NG tube/NBM		
Management includes Abdominal x-ray		
Management includes erect Chest x-ray		
Management includes blood tests including group and save		
Management includes analgesia		
Appropriately refers to surgical team and critical care		
Correctly describes abdominal x-ray findings		
Examiner's Global Mark	/5	
Actor / Helper's Global Mark	/5	
Total Station Mark	/30	

Learning points

- The ABCDE approach is crucial in a scenario like this, especially reassessing the patient after intervention or a change (e.g. patient vomits).

- Acute bowel obstruction can lead to profound hypovolaemic shock requiring IV fluids and critical care support. If there is blood loss early consideration of blood products is prudent

- Expose patient to look for causes including scars (previous surgery), herniae, intraabdominal masses, and don't forget PR exam.

9. Haematemesis

Candidate's Instructions

You are the foundation doctor working in the Emergency Department. A 78-year-old female has been brought in with haematemesis. This patient needs to be seen as a priority as there are concerns that she may need prompt intervention. Currently the patient states she has been vomiting up fresh red blood.

Your consultant asks you to do an A-E assessment on this patient and implement appropriate initial interventions, then report back to them with your findings and any concerns.

Examiner's Instructions

A 78-year-old female has been brought to the Emergency department with haematemesis. The patient states she has been vomiting up fresh red blood.

The foundation doctor in the emergency medicine team has been asked to do an A to E assessment and implement appropriate initial interventions.

Observe the candidate doing the initial introduction and history, then assess their A – E approach of examination, investigations and interventions using the mark scheme below. The candidate will need some feedback about the assessment they are carrying out which are as follows.

These are only to be given if the candidate specifically asks for each one:

A   Airway patent but patient has fresh red blood stains around mouth. Suction can be used to remove blood in the mouth

B   RR 24, Sats 100%. Bilateral equal chest wall movement, normal percussion and normal breath sounds on auscultation.

C   HR 105 Regular, bilateral radial pulses present. Central CRT<2, warm peripheries, slightly clammy. BP 110/73.

If candidate asks for a VBG - pH 7.34, Hb 110, Electrolytes normal, Lactate 1.8, HCO_3 22.1. Bloods tests to be sent should include FBC, Group and saves, clotting and U&E's

D   GCS 15, PEARL. BM 7.6.

E   Temp 35.0, no rash, no evidence of CLD. Tender epigastrium.

PR exam - black stool, no fresh red blood with normal anal tone. No haemorrhoids.

At the end of the assessment, ask the candidate to summarise their A-E assessment and ask whether there is anything else they'd like to do?

Actor's Instructions

You are a 78-year-old female who has been brought to the Emergency department because you are vomiting fresh red blood. A doctor has been asked to see you and assess you immediately as you are very worried about what is going on.

You woke up this morning with a pain in your upper central stomach, 5/10 on a pain score, which felt like indigestion or reflux. No radiation to anywhere. Then about an hour ago you vomited up fresh red blood, about a bowl full, with some clots. You have had 3 small vomits of fresh red blood since then. You are feeling slightly dizzy now but no shortness of breath, chest pain or palpitations. You have not passed out. Other than today you have not noticed any problems - your bowels are open regularly, no blood noticed in your stool but you haven't checked really. You haven't had any problems with passing urine and your abdomen doesn't feel bloated. You haven't noticed any weight loss recently or night sweats and have felt relatively well apart from a few joint aches and pains. You have been eating and drinking well.

You have a previous medical history of a bilateral knee arthritis - this has been getting worse recently so you are awaiting knee replacement and have been started on naproxen until then. Other than that you suffer with mild acid reflux and high blood pressure.

Your current medications are Naproxen 250mg four times a day, gaviscon when you need it and amlodipine 10mg a day. You have no known drug allergies. You have no other medical history or surgical history.

Your have no family history of any cancer. Your mum died of a heart attack aged 82.

You currently live alone and are fully independent. You do not smoke and very rarely drink- maybe a tipple of sherry at Christmas. You are retired and a fairly active golfer.

You are very worried about what is causing this and are worried you may die if you lose too much blood. This makes you quite upset and agitated.

Mark Scheme - Haematemesis

Task	Achieved	Not-Achieved
Washes hands, introduces self.		
Clarifies whom they are speaking to and begins to build rapport with patient.		
Very brief and focused HPC, PMH, D&A, SH plus explanation of assessment to patient		
Airway - look, listen, feel. Check patency		
Airway interventions - High flow oxygen + manoeuvres, insert airways and suction as required.		
Breathing – RR and Sats.		
Chest wall movement, percussion, auscultation. CXR if necessary		
Circulation assessment- HR, BP. ECG if required.		
Central CRT , Radial pulse, peripheries.		
Circulation interventions- 2 large bore cannula. Consider IVF.		
Bloods for FBC/U&E's, Clotting, LFTs and G&S plus VBG.		
Cross match suitable units for patient- discuss with lab.		
Catheter and fluid balance chart		
Disability - check BG. Assess GCS and pupils.		
Exposure – Check temperature. Check for abdo tenderness signs of chronic liver disease.		
Do PR examination		
Exposure intervention- Warm up as required and other urgent interventions.		
Competently able to summarises the A-E assessment and interventions for patient		
Knows limitations and would call for help/refer a.s.a.p. during scenario		
Works with the patient in a professional yet caring manner to keep them calm and enable treatment.		
Examiner's Global Mark	/5	
Actor / Helper's Global Mark	/5	
Total Station Mark	/30	

Learning points

- If the patient is initially haemodynamically unstable the first action must be to do an A to E assessment with appropriate interventions along the way- two large bore cannula, bloods, venous blood gas and Group and Save. Always call for help.

- There are two scoring systems for an upper GI bleed. The Glasgow-Blatchford bleeding score (GBS): this is a screening tool which can assess which place is safest for the patient to be managed and whether they will need any interventions such as blood transfusion or endoscopy.

- The Rockall risk scoring system: this scoring system assesses risk factors during acute upper GI bleed to predict mortality. There is an initial score prior to endoscopy and a full score given after endoscopy is completed. Any score of 3 or above will have a higher mortality and risk of rebleed. In the ED a Blatchford score can be used to to stratify low risk patients for outpatient management.

10. ACS and heart failure

Candidate's Instructions

You are the foundation doctor in the Emergency Department resus area and have been asked to see a 65-year-old man who has been brought in by ambulance complaining of left sided chest pain and shortness of breath.

The senior registrar in ED asks you to undertake the initial structured assessment. You are asked to report your findings and management plan at each stage to the team. You have 6 minutes to complete your assessment.

After 6 minutes the examiner will stop you and ask for a diagnosis. A competent nurse is assisting you.

Examiner's Instructions

A 65-year-old man has been brought into the ED resus via ambulance complaining of left sided chest pain and shortness of breath.

The foundation doctor has been asked to undertake the initial structured assessment of the patient and feed back his findings and management plan at each stage. Please provide the candidate with the following values as requested

A   Patent

B   On auscultation-fine creps and fine wheeze bi-basally
RR 26, sats 91% RA, sats 98% on 15L via non-rebreathe mask

ABG results- on their way
CXR- upper lobe diversion, fine patchy shadowing both bases, Kerley B lines

C   HR 90, BP 100/60, CRT 2s, T36.8
     The patient appears clammy, grey and sweaty
     ECG- widespread ST depression, sinus rhythm
     HS- regular, no added sounds

D   BM 12.3

E   No abnormalities

As the candidate reaches E, the nurse informs them that the patient is no longer breathing. Ask the candidate their immediate escalation plan.

At 6 minutes stop the scenario and ask the candidate to give his impression of the diagnosis.

Actor's Instructions

You are a 65-year-old man brought into ED resus via ambulance. You called 999 as you experienced sudden onset left sided chest pain and shortness of breath.

A - You are able to talk and respond to the candidate, albeit breathlessly.

B - You are breathing fast and shallowly. You feel much worse when you are   laying flat.

C - You feel sweaty, clammy and nauseous.

D - You are fully conscious and aware of who and where you are.

E - When the candidate reaches this stage you should stop responding as you have now lost consciousness

Mark scheme

Task	Achieved	Not Achieved
Introduces self, washes hands and checks patient identity		
Explicitly comments on patient airway patency		
Starts 15L oxygen via non-rebreathe mask		
Comments on respiratory effort		
Asks for oxygen saturations and RR		
Percusses and auscultates the chest		
Requests ABG and CXR		
Asks for HR, BP, Temp, urinary catheter, ECG and cardiac monitoring, blood tests including troponin		
Assess radial pulse, CRT, auscultates for heart sounds		
Starts ACS protocol- Morphine, Oxygen, Nitrates, Aspirin, Clopidogrel, mentions doses and routes. -		
Comments on rational for holding IVF and starting IV furosemide.		
Comments on referral to cardiology/cath lab		
Explicitly mentions GCS or AVPU		
Examines pupils		
Asks for BM		
Explicitly mentions examining the rest of the body		
States pull crash button and place 2222 arrest call		
Correctly identifies diagnosis of ACS		
Flash pulmonary oedema		
Demonstrates systematic ABCDE approach		
Examiner's Global Mark	/5	
Actor / Helper's Global Mark	/5	
Total Station Mark	/30	

Learning Points

- Being familiar with utilising an A to E approach in the assessment and management of the sick patient. Remember to treat each finding before moving on to the next step.

- Be familiar with the treatment of ACS - MONAC

  Morphine sulphate 10mg PO or 5mg IV
  Oxygen- high flow via non-rebreath mask
  Nitrates- 1 puff S/L GTN spray (400mcg)
  Aspirin- 300mg PO
  Clopidogrel- 300mg PO

- Communicating your assessment, impression and plan of the patient is key to getting your patient treated promptly. In the exam scenario you must get into the habit of describing your findings out loud and asking for observations and treatments in order to get your marks, a bit like a driving test. In the clinical setting, this same approach will ensure you and your team are all on the same page, ensuring treatments are started in a timely manner.

11. Sepsis 6 and SIRS

Candidate's Instructions

You are the foundation doctor in the Emergency Department. The ED sister has informed you that a patient has spiked a temperature and has a high pulse rate, pain in her abdomen and some dysuria. She is a direct referral from GP and has not yet been reviewed by a doctor. Please review this patient and perform a focused examination.

After 6 minutes the examiner will stop you and ask you to summarise back your findings, suggest your differential diagnoses and your initial management plan.

Examiner's instructions

This 22-year-old woman has been admitted to the Emergency Department with a urinary tract infection. She starts to have a fever and the nurse has found her to have a high pulse rate of 130 beats per minute. Her blood pressure is 100/80.

She is triggering on the National Early Warning Score (NEWS) having a systemic inflammatory response syndrome caused by the urine infection. Together this means that she is suffering from sepsis.

The candidate will do an A to E assessment of the patient. The actor playing a nurse in this situation will provide the vital signs of the patient to the candidate.

At 6 minutes or before if the candidate has finished then you should ask the candidate to summarise their findings, provide a differential diagnosis and suggest a management plan.

Actors instructions

Patient:

You will allow the candidate to examine you. You will have had lower abdominal pain for the last 3 days, pain when passing urine and have had increased frequency of passing urine. Try and only explain these symptoms if they ask. The pain has now moved up to the left side of your abdomen and to your kidney. You have been having high temperatures but have not measured them and have been shivering and shaking. You currently feel cold and sweaty. You feel your heart is racing.

Nurse:

You are a senior nurse and will provide the doctor with the patient's vital signs when requested and put on the appropriate monitoring.

Sats 99% on room air
P130
BP100/80
Cap refill 3s
Temp 38.6

If asked you will say that you can organise the taking of some blood cultures and a venous blood gas. The full blood count taken when the patient arrived showed the white cell count was 13.

Mark Scheme: Sepsis

Task:	Achieved	Not Achieved
Washes hands and introduces self to patient and nurse		
Elicits a focused history		
Confirms Airway is patent		
Asks for oxygen saturation and respiratory rate		
Asks to give high flow oxygen		
Auscultates chest		
Feels for Pulse asks for blood pressure		
Tests the patients capillary refill time		
Requests IV cannula		
Requests blood tests FBC, U&Es, Venous blood gas and blood cultures		
Asks for an intravenous fluid bolus 10ml/kg		
Examines the patient's abdomen		
Elicits kidney pain		
Establishes the patient's Glasgow coma score		
Asks for a blood sugar level		
Asks to measure patient's urine output or asks to insert a catheter		
Suggests appropriate differential diagnosis		
Sepsis from kidney infection		
Suggest an appropriate management plan		
Mentions the instigation of the sepsis six and states to give antibiotics ASAP		
Examiners Global Mark	/5	
Actor/Helpers Global Mark	/5	
Total Station Mark	/30	

Learning points:

- Sepsis is a common presentation for patients in hospital and the speed with which it is treated is very important. The sepsis trust stipulates certain time goals for each part of the process e.g. give the sepsis 6 within one hour from suspicion of sepsis.

- Know your sepsis six. An aid memoire is 'give 3, take 2 and monitor 1!'. Give; high flow oxygen, Iv fluid bolus and Iv antibiotics. Take; iv blood cultures and VBG for a lactate. Monitor urine output.

-

- If the lactate level is higher than 4mmol/kg the patient will need critical care review and possible ITU admission. Observing trends in the lactate can be a method of knowing if your interventions are working.

-

12. Diabetic Ketoacidosis

Candidate's instructions

You are the foundation doctor working in the Emergency Department. A 24-year-old university student has just been brought into the ED with profuse vomiting for the past 12 hours. He had been at a barbeque with friends yesterday enjoying a few beers and some food. He had gone to bed early after 'not feeling quite right'. He thought he might have had a few too many drinks but he awoke at 2am with abdominal pain and perfuse vomiting. You have a nurse with you to help.

An arterial blood gas has been done:

pH 7.22
PCO2 3.2
PO2 17
Bicarbonate 5.8
Base excess -25
Na 147
K 6.2
Glucose 32
Lactate 6

Take a focused history from the patient and perform an initial assessment. Decide on a likely diagnosis, discuss this with the nurse and give a plan for any urgent investigations and treatment required, along with treatment goals. Ensure you complete the fluid prescription chart if any fluids are required.

Actor's instructions

You are a 22-year-old university student who has been brought into the ED with a 12-hour history of abdominal pain and vomiting. A doctor is going to examine you and try to make an initial diagnosis and initiate a management plan.

You were diagnosed with type 1 diabetes when you were 19. You initially found your insulin difficult to manage but now you find it much easier, although you do occasionally forget to take it. You have not needed any emergency admissions since your diagnosis and see your GP regularly for a medication review. You had your appendix removed age 7. You are otherwise entirely fit and well.

Drug history

Insuman rapid 9 units before breakfast
Insuman rapid 9 units before lunch
Novorapid 10 units before dinner
Levemir 10 units before dinner
No known drug allergies.

You were at a friend's BBQ yesterday and spent all day in the sunshine drinking beer. You're a vegetarian and there wasn't really any vegetarian options so you didn't eat much - for this reason you haven't taken any insulin since 9 am yesterday (it is now 2 pm). Do not volunteer this information unless directly asked.

You started to feel a bit unwell at 7 pm and went home. You felt nauseated and had a mild stomach ache but think this was because you had been out in the sun all day and had drank 5 bottles of beer which is quite a lot for you. You went to bed but awoke at 2 am feeling very sick and with abdominal pain. You have been profusely vomiting since (>30 times). You are vomiting yellow/green fluid with no evidence of blood. Your abdominal pain is generalised with no focus, a constant cramping sensation that does not radiate anywhere and has been mild throughout (3/10). Your bowel habits and stool are normal. You were initially passing urine often but are now passing very little.

You appear to be in mild discomfort and have a rapid breathing pattern. You are feeling drowsy and only provide the information outlined above if directly asked. Your abdomen is mildly tender when pressed. No focal area of pain.

Nurse's instructions

You are a band 5 nurse so have a good level of experience and can independently place monitoring and fulfill the requests the doctor has.

Examiner's Instructions

The doctor has been asked to see a 24-year-old insulin dependent diabetic patient who has just been brought into the emergency department with a 12-hour history of vomiting and abdominal pain. The patient had been out in the sun all of the previous day and had a moderate amount of alcohol. He had not eaten much all day and so he did not take his insulin. He has DKA.

The candidate has been asked to take a focused history - this should centre on the presenting complaint and the events leading up to this presentation. Salient points from his medical history should also be covered (diagnosis of diabetes) as well as his drug history.

The candidate has been asked to do an initial assessment of the patient, this should consist of an A-E approach. As the patient is examined and monitoring is placed the following is found:

A - Patent

B - Respiratory rate 24, Saturations 100% on room air, Chest is clear with bilateral air entry

C - A little cool peripherally, Heart rate 117, Blood pressure 120/67, ECG sinus. No abnormality. Normal T waves.

D - GCS 15 but very tired and only occasionally answering questions fully Blood glucose 32

E - No obvious injuries, No rashes, Temperature 36.8, Abdomen is mildly tender to palpation. No focus. No guarding. Normal bowel sounds.

The candidate has been asked to identify a likely diagnosis and outline to the nurse any urgent investigations and management. Although they may wish to rule out other causes of the patient's presentation they should identify DKA as the most likely diagnosis and focus their answer on this.

Investigations	Management	Treatment goals (60 min)
Urine dip to confirm diagnosis	Fluids - 0.9% saline without potassium. 1L over 1-2 hours to begin replacement. Fluid bolus not required.	Restore circulating volume (reduce heart rate)
ECG	Insulin - Fixed rate IV insulin infusion at approximately 0.1 units/Kg/ hour.	Reduce blood ketone concentration by 0.5 mmol/L/hour
CXR	Treatment of hyperkalaemia	Reduce blood glucose by 3-5 mmol/L/hour
Blood tests - FBC, renal profile, serum osmolarity, lab glucose, serum ketones. Allow others if well justified.	Critical care referral	Maintain K+ between 4-5mmol/L

Do not award marks for:
Venous/ arterial gas as this has been made available in the question.
Sodium bicarbonate as it is not considered mainstay treatment.

One minute before the end of the station: Stop the candidate and ask them to confirm what they think the likely diagnosis is (if not already stated) and to name two potentially life-threatening complications of DKA.

Mark Scheme

Task	Achieved	Not Achieved
Introduces themselves to the patient, establishes need for consult and seeks consent		
Introduces themselves to nurse and establishes experience		
Washes hands		
Requests monitoring		
Takes a focused history from patient		
Establishes airway is patient and not compromised		
Listens to the chest. Notes Raised respiratory rate		
Notes they are tachycardic		
Notes their GCS and that they are drowsy. Blood glucose is available.		
Abdominal examination. Checks for injuries and rashes.		
Requests an ECG - notes concerns regarding potassium		
Requests urinary/serum ketones to confirm diagnosis		
Obtains IV access		
Recognises DKA as likely diagnosis		
Initiates fluid therapy at appropriate rate		
Prescribes fluid therapy correctly		
Initiates/ notes the need for insulin infusion		
Communicates well with nursing colleague throughout		
Sets monitoring requirement for nurse and initial therapy goals		
Can identify 2 potential complication of DKA		
Examiner's Global Mark	/5	
Actor / Helper's Global Mark	/5	
Total Station Mark	/30	

Learning points

- DKA is a potentially life threatening complication of diabetes and as doctors we need to be aware that it is easy to 'forget the glucose'. On an A-E approach D is for disability and should also be for *'don't forget the glucose'*.

- Insulin is essential in the management of DKA, however, dehydration is often more immediately life threatening and thus takes priority. Patients can require remarkably large quantities of fluid to restore their circulating volume. This can risk causing sudden shifts between fluid compartments and can lead to the potentially fatal complication of cerebral oedema.

- Electrolyte disturbance is another important complication to be aware of, as is hypoglycaemia! Therapy therefore requires a careful approach and regular reassessment. Local DKA protocols vary with regards to fluid resuscitation, insulin infusions and potassium control and it is always worth checking them.

Reference

Joint British Diabetes Societies Inpatient Care Group. The Management of Diabetic Ketoacidosis in Adults. March 2010

13. Status Epilepticus

Candidate's Instructions:

A 25-year-old man is brought into the Emergency Department having a generalised tonic-clonic seizure, which started 15 minutes ago. The paramedic team have been unable to secure IV access but have administered one dose of rectal diazepam 10 minutes ago. The patient has no past medical history and does not take any regular medication.

You are the foundation doctor on the acute medical take and have been called to the Emergency Department to manage this patient. You have an experienced staff nurse with you to help.

After 6 minutes the examiner will stop you and ask you to summarise back your findings, suggest your differential diagnoses and your management plan from here on.

Examiner's Instructions:

A 25-year-old man is brought into the Emergency Department having a generalised tonic-clonic seizure that started 15 minutes ago. The paramedic team have been unable to secure IV access but have administered one dose of rectal diazepam 10 minutes ago.

The foundation doctor has been called to manage this patient. If asked by the candidate please provide the following information:

The medical emergency team/senior help is on their way to assist you.
On initial assessment:

Patient is having a tonic-clonic seizure

A – jaw clenched, foaming at the mouth, gurgling noises from upper airway.
Once airway suctioned and nasopharyngeal airway inserted, noises from upper airway improve.
B – shallow breathing, RR 30, oxygen saturations 88% in room air, increased to 100% on high flow oxygen, clear lung fields on auscultation
C – pulse rate 120, blood pressure 140/88, warm peripheries, capillary refill time <2sec
D – GCS 3/15, blood sugar 3.5
E – no rashes, temperature 37.0

You may speed up intervals between drugs being administered and ask the candidate what they would like to do next during the scenario however no other prompts please.

After 6 minutes, if not done so, please prompt the candidate for a diagnosis and ask the candidate to summarise a handover of the case to an ICU colleague.

Actor's Instructions:

You are a staff nurse in the Emergency Department. You are able to assist the candidate and you know where all the equipment is kept. You are not able to perform tasks unless clearly instructed to by the candidate.

Mark Scheme

Task	Achieved	Not Achieved
Appropriate introduction and task allocation to team members		
Calls early for senior help		
Ensures all members of the team wear appropriate PPE		
Appropriate assessment of patient's airway		
Makes attempt to suction patient's mouth and upper airway		
States would use airway adjunct (ie. nasopharyngeal airway) to maintain airway		
Commences high flow oxygen - 15L via non-rebreathe mask		
Assessment of breathing - RR, oxygen saturations, auscultation, percussion		
Assessment of circulation - BP, HR, capillary refill time		
States would like to gain IV/IO access and send appropriate samples to laboratory		
Explicitly states would like to check BM		
States would like to commence IV/IO dextrose (50ml of 50% solution)		
Assessment of neurological status		
Adequately exposes patient		
Makes diagnosis of status epilepticus		
States would administer IV/IO lorazepam or Diazepam		
States no response to benzodiazepines so commences loading with phenytoin		
Inform anaesthetist/ICU and prepares for intubation		
Appropriate handover to ICU colleague when they arrive		
Demonstrates systematic A-E assessment		
Examiner's Global Mark	/5	
Actor / Helper's Global Mark	/5	
Total Station Mark	/30	

Learning points:

- Status epilepticus is a medical emergency and is defined as continuous seizure activity lasting more than 30 minutes, or repeated tonic–clonic convulsions occurring over a 30 minutes period without recovery of consciousness between each convulsion. Any seizure however that lasts more than 5 minutes needs to be treated as status epilepticus as termination of the seizure can became increasingly difficult.

- The first line of treatment for a seizure is benzodiazepines. Common preparations include rectal diazepam, buccal midazolam or intravenous lorazepam. If the first dose does not terminate the seizure within 5 minutes, administer a second dose.

- On-going assessment of the patient whilst having a seizure includes a neurological examination to look for a focal intra-cranial lesion and to consider hypoglycaemia as both can cause seizures or as a result of prolonged seizure activity.

14. Hyperkalaemia

Candidate's Instructions

You are a foundation doctor working in the resuscitation area of the emergency department when a new patient arrives. A 62-year-old lady has been referred in by the GP with 'abnormal blood results'.

Her past medical history includes congestive cardiac failure, chronic kidney disease, hypertension and gout.

Perform an initial assessment A through E assessment correcting any abnormalities as you go.

Examiner's Instructions

This 62-year-old lady had a set of blood tests at the GP this morning. The GP has requested she attend the emergency department immediately as the plasma potassium came back at 7.1mmol/l.

The student should perform a systematic A to E assessment.

A - Patent

B – Equal air entry, Clear chest, RR 18, Sats 98% on Air

C – HR-84, BP 118/75, Cap refill < 2. The venous gas results show a potassium of 7.1mmol/l and a PH 7.35 with all other results within normal limits. The student should request an ECG. They must be handed a good example of the changes seen in hyperkalaemia.

Allow the student to interpret the ECG, without prompting. They must identify that this is a medical emergency and treat appropriately. Tall tented T waves, with loss of P waves and widening of the QRS are common features to look out for,

D - GCS 15, BM 5.1

E – General muscle ache, No signs of haemorrhage

Actor's Instructions:

You are a 62 year old lady with a past medical history includes congestive cardiac failure, chronic kidney disease, hypertension and gout. You have blood tests four times a year and your kidney function has always been relatively stable according to the consultants.

You have not had any change in medications but have been unwell for 5 days with diarrhoea and vomiting and hardly been able to keep anything but small sips of water down. You have continued to take your medication though as you know you should never miss them.

Yesterday you had 'an unusual beating in the chest' and general muscle pains so the GP sent you for a blood test. You had a phone call from GP surgery asking you to go to the hospital urgently as one of the blood markers was raised. You have been taken to the resus room and a juior doctor is about to review you.

Mark Scheme: Hyperkalaemia

Task	Achieved	Not Achieved
Introduces themselves, consents and washes hands		
A – looks for signs of obstruction, attaches oxygen		
B - counts respiratory rate		
Attaches arterial saturations probe		
Inspects chest expansion & checks position of trachea		
Percusses chest & Auscultates thorax		
C – Colour, temperature, capillary refill time		
Comments on heart rate and blood pressure		
Looks for signs of haemorrhage		
Inserts IV access and takes blood including VBG		
Requests ECG		
Correctly identifies changes associated with high K^+		
Confirms with VBG		
Attach continuous cardiac monitoring		
Gives: 10mls of 10% Calcium chloride or calcium gluconate		
Insulin Dextrose – 10 units actrapid in 120mls 20% dextrose		
Suggests 0.9% Sodium chloride infusion		
Considers salbutamol nebulizer if delay in insulin dextrose		
D and E - Checks GCS and Blood glucose		
Mentions the possibility of dialysis or haemofiltration if hyperkalaemia refractory to Insulin dextrose.		
Examiner's Global Mark	/5	
Actor / Helper's Global Mark	/5	
Total Station Mark	/30	

Learning Points

- Classic causes of hyperkalemia include; Insulin insufficiency as insulin drives potassium intracellularly or the inability to excrete potassium through the kidneys.

- In cardiac arrest, continue with resuscitation until potassium normalized. Once ROSC achieved, continue insulin and dextrose until the repeat blood gases demonstrate an improvement.

- Consider dialysis or haemofiltration for hyperkalaemia that is resistant to routine medical therapy,

15. Shortness of breath : DVT/PE

Candidate's instructions

You are the foundation doctor in the Emergency Department. You have been asked to see this 24-year-old lady who has presented with shortness of breath. Please take a full history.

After 6 minutes the examiner will stop you and ask you to summarise back your findings, suggest your differential diagnoses and your initial management plan.

Examiner's instructions

This 28-year-old woman has presented to the ED with shortness of breath. The foundation doctor has been asked to take a history with a view to discussing the differential diagnosis and further management plan.

She has a PE with a history consistent with a DVT as well. She has returned from New Zealand two days ago and takes the oral contraceptive pill.

This station allows the candidate to demonstrate their ability to take a history of shortness of breath and chest pain.

They should specifically ask for VTE risk factors. There is a cardiac family history which should be elicited both as part of this history and to establish that she is most worried about having a heart attack. There is a personal history of anxiety, which should be touched on, but not explored too deeply. While a panic attack is part of the differential, a PE should be excluded.

Stop the candidate at 6 minutes to discuss their further management plan. This should include as a minimum examination, observations, blood tests and a chest x-ray.

If they are able to identify PE as the most likely diagnosis on the basis of the history, tell them that this is correct and continue the discussion. If not tell them that the patient has a PE and continue from there.

The candidate should be able to discuss scoring systems for a PE. They should be aware of the Well's score and how to apply the score in clinical practice. Without further observations the Well's score cannot be calculated but from the history alone she is sufficiently high risk to warrant further imaging. The candidate should be aware that a d-dimer is only of use in low risk patients and that a negative d-dimer in the context of a high risk patient is insufficient to exclude a PE.

Tell them that the patient does have a PE. Ask them what their treatment plan would be? They should know that the patient needs a low molecular weight heparin followed by warfarin or a novel oral anti-coagulant. Ask whether the candidate knows of another treatment in the context of a life-threatening PE. They should be aware that thrombolysis is an option but the criteria for thrombolysis is not required information.

Actor's instructions

On your way to work this morning you noticed that you were short of breath, which is unusual for you. You didn't think much of it until you were climbing the stairs on the way into the office and it became worse and was associated with some left sided chest pain. It is this that is worrying you most and prompted you to come into the ED.

You have had a slight cough that is not productive since yesterday. You have not coughed up any blood. You do not feel like you've had any fevers or sweats. The pain was sharp in nature and when questioned tell the candidate that it is worse when you took a deep breath in. It did not radiate anywhere. At it's worst it was 7/10 but at rest and at the moment you don't feel any pain. You are having some difficulty talking in long sentences. You have not taken any painkillers. Both your shortness of breath and chest pain are worse when you exert yourself.

Reveal these details only if asked directly:
You came back from holiday in New Zealand 2 weeks ago. You noticed some swelling of your legs on the flight but since being back you left leg has returned to normal but your right is still swollen and is starting to become painful.

Your other medical complaints consist of only anxiety for which you take an antidepressant. You have never had any operations. You are also taking the oral contraceptive pill. You have no allergies.

If directly asked about your family history explain that your dad had a heart attack three months ago and you are very worried that this might be a heart attack. He is 48 years old. There is no family history of DVT or PE.

You work in a property development firm which is mostly behind a desk. You exercise regularly, gave up smoking 3 years ago and drink socially 1-2 times per week. You have never taken any recreational drugs.

Mark Scheme: Shortness of breath : DVT/PE

Task	Achieved	Not Achieved
Introduces self, washes hands and checks identity		
Elicits history from patient in a concise manner		
Asks questions to explore the possibility of other cases of shortness of breath: cough, fevers, exacerbating and relieving factors, associated chest pain.		
Asks about past medical history (previous history of clots or varicose veins)		
Asks family history (previous history of clots or sudden death or inherited factor disorders)		
Asks about drug history (anticoagulants or COCP)		
Asks about social history (smoking and recent travel)		
Asks about specific VTE risk factors: recent immobility, operations		
Asks about pregnancy or LMP		
Elicits concern about heart problems after her father's heart attack		
Reacts to patient's concerns in an empathic and non-judgemental manner		
Is able to summarise findings		
Generates a reasonable differential diagnosis including respiratory and cardiac complaints		
Discusses the need for basic blood tests and knows to consider a d-dimer in this context		
Can discuss the use of a d-dimer in risk assessment for VTE		
Discusses the need for imaging. Chest x-ray at least and knows to consider CTPA or V/Q		
Is able to give at least one scoring system for assessing PE risk.		
Identifies that this patient is likely high risk for a PE.		
Is aware of the need for anticoagulation with LMWH followed by warfarin		
Is aware of thrombolysis as a management option in a life threatening PE.		
Examiner's Global Mark	/5	
Actor / Helper's Global Mark	/5	
Total Station Mark	/30	

Learning points

- Scoring systems for a PE include the popular Well's score, the Geneva score and the Pulmonary Embolism Severity Index or PESI score.

- A d-dimer is useful to exclude a PE in the low risk patient. If a patient is low risk and has a negative d-dimer they are unlikely to have a PE. If they are low risk with a raised d-dimer they may have a PE but the test may be raised for a variety of other reasons. If they are high risk they should have further investigations for a PE by way of a CTPA (or V/Q in certain cases) even if their d-dimer is normal making it an unnecessary test.

- Other causes of a raised d-dimer include: Aortic dissection, malignancy, sepsis, acute coronary syndromes, upper GI bleeds, disseminated intravascular coagulation (DIC), stroke and AF.

16. Atrial Fibrillation

Candidate's Instructions:

You are the foundation doctor in the Emergency Department and have been asked to see a 82 year old lady who has been brought by her daughter. She has been complaining that for the last 3 days she has been feeling her heart beating fast in her chest with bouts of chest pain. Her daughter has brought her to hospital today as she complained about feeling dizzy and had a "funny spell".

After 6 minutes the examiner will stop you and ask you to summarise back your findings, suggest your differential diagnoses and your initial management plan.

Examiner's Instructions:

This 82-year-old lady has presented to the Emergency Department with palpitations and paroxysmal atrial fibrillation.

The candidate should do the following:

- Take a clear history from the patient
- Ask about the symptoms of palpitation, how long it has lasted for, has she had symptoms of this before, how long did each episode of palpitations last for
- In regards to her chest pain, where was the pain located, what was the chest pain like, how long did it last for, is she currently in pain, any aggravating or relieving factors, any other symptoms at the time of the chest pain (sweatiness, SOB, etc)
- Any other past medical history including previous cardiac issues
- Drug history and other medications
- Social history if she smokes or drinks heavily and who does she live at home with

At 6 minutes, please stop the candidate at whatever point they are at in the history and ask them to summarise their findings and what differentials they can decipher from their history.

Ask the candidate
"What investigations would you think about doing for this patient?"

Appropriate answers:

- ECG → Show an ECG showing Atrial fibrillation. Candidate should be able to recognize AF on an ECG (irregular rhythm with absence of p waves)
- Bloods include troponin → 25 (candidate should know to ask for a repeat troponin)

- Septic screen (including CXR or urine dip) → Any signs of infection
- Checking for electrolyte abnormalities

Advise the candidate

"Your patient is stable and is very keen to go home. On repeat ECG, her AF appears to be ongoing but rate controlled and not fast, her bloods and her septic screen have come back normal. Please discuss with the patient what is causing her symptoms and what follow up management and treatment she requires"

Candidate should know the following:

- CHADSVASC2 score to decide if patient requires anticoagulation and what is most appropriate.
- Should explain briefly without use of jargon what atrial fibrillation is and the risks that can occur with it.
- As she has co-morbidities and is >75 with acute AF, she requires anti-coagulation (with warfarin) and candidate should advise patient that she will require an outpatient echo and potentially cardioversion in the future.

Actor's Instructions

You are an 82-year-old lady who has been having episodes of shortness of breath with associated feelings of your heart beating rapidly in your chest. It has been coming and going for the last 3 days. You've not had anything like this before. You became concerned this evening and told your daughter as it stopped you from sleeping.

With the feeling of your heart beating in your chest, over the last 24 hours, you have also had some chest pain which has caused you some worry. You haven't had problems with your heart before but have slightly raised blood pressure. You do not take medication for it as the medications can sometimes make you feel dizzy.

Your daughter called for an ambulance this evening as you were unable to sleep because of your heart beating in your chest. You had some accompanying chest pain on the left side of the chest that felt like 'tightness' but eased off by itself after 2-3 minutes. However you also had a dizzy spell requiring you to sit down. You deny any infective symptoms.

You think it's just your old age and do not understand what all the fuss is about and would just like to go home to bed. You REFUSE point blank to stay in hospital. You live with your daughter, after all, who can care for you.

You have a past medical history of reflux, high blood pressure, high cholesterol, "may have had a mini stroke but it resolved by itself so I didn't really worry about it"

You are technically on bisoprolol 2.5mg OD but do not take it regularly. You also take Simvastatin and omeprazole. There are no known drug allergies.

You are an ex-smoker who quit 3 years ago. You live with your daughter and walk around with a frame. You don't drink alcohol except on your birthday and at christmas.

When discussing the atrial fibrillation, keep repeating "but my heart has always been fine. I don't understand how this has happened. I don't want to take any medicines".

When warfarin is mentioned "but that is rat poison. Some of my friends have taken that and they say they had bad side effects from it. Is this true?"

When investigations are mentioned, refuse to stay in hospital overnight. Once the investigations have come back normal and the patient has been discussed with a senior colleague they can be discharged home with outpatient follow up.

Mark Scheme: Atrial Fibrillation

Task	Achieved	Not Achieved
Introduces self and washes hands		
Clarifies who they are speaking to		
Elicits history in a concise manner		
Asks about palpitations: length of time, other symptoms, previous episodes		
Asks about chest pain: SOCRATES		
Ask about past medical history		
Asks about drug history & compliance		
Enquires about social situation: carers, mobilising, smoking, drinking		
Performs an ECG		
Septic screen: Urine dip, CXR, bloods		
Troponin and repeat troponin		
Outpatient → BNP, anticoagulation clinic follow up, echo		
Explains atrial fibrillation – simply, no jargon		
Explains CHADSVASC2 score and need for anticoagulation		
Explains need for follow up		
If concerned about unsafe discharge, discuss with senior colleague		
Explain indication to patient for warfarin		
Doesn't collude with parent		
Remains calm		
Non judgmental approach		
Examiner's Global Mark	/5	
Actor / Helper's Global Mark	/5	
Total Station Mark	/30	

Learning Points

- In scenarios like this one, you need to be concise and quite efficient with your questioning to ensure you get the information you need in a short space of time, to come up with a differential diagnosis, and a management plan.

- Guidelines and scoring systems are very useful tools to help in deciding management plans for patients. Using evidence based medicine should be the basis for all decision making where possible, and gives the clinician validity in their recommendations.

- Ensure patient safety at all times. If you are unsure if the patient should be allowed to go home because they could be unsafe then discuss the case with a senior asap (both in real life and in a scenario like this).

17. Carbon monoxide

Candidate's Instructions

You are the foundation doctor working in the Emergency Department majors area. You are asked to see a patient who felt dizzy at home and has collapsed in front of their house whilst leaving to go shopping. They recovered quickly but still feel unwell. Please take a focused history and then perform a rapid A to E examination.

After 6 minutes the examiner will stop you and ask you to summarise back your findings, suggest your differential diagnoses, the investigations required and your initial management plan.

Examiner's Instructions

After 6 minutes, please stop the candidate and ask which relevant investigations you would like and which treatment would be first line to commence. Ask about indications for hyperbaric oxygen therapy.

If asked, the patient's examination, observations and ABG are as follows:

A: patent

B: Chest clear, SpO2 97%, RR 18

ABG: pH 7.25, PO2 12, CO2 3.0, SpO2 82%, Lac 5.0 HCO3 18.2, BE - 7.4.

C: BP 110/60 Pulse 95.

At this stage, the candidate should ask for a carbon monoxide level, which is 15%.

ECG: Sinus arrhythmia with PVE (premature ventricular ectopics), T wave inversion across chest leads.

If asked for MetHb, it is 0.6%

D: GCS 15/15

E: Afebrile

Urinalysis: Protein ++, Glucose +

If there is time you can ask about how the half life of carbon monoxide compares when breathing room air to 100% O2.

Actor's Instructions

You are a 40-year-old single mother who is self employed as a building surveyor. You have a 10-year-old son who also lives with you. You have been fit and healthy over the past years. You do not take any regular medication. You do not smoke, but drink a moderate amount of alcohol.

Since the winter started you have been struggling with work at home. You frequently get dizzy spells and are easily fatigued. You have had a headache, usually every day, for about 1 month. The headache is a dull, constant ache at the front of your head. After a long day you sometimes get palpitations and lately you have found it hard to concentrate. You have put these symptoms down to working too hard and taking care of your son.

Your son has been quite well but in the last few weeks has often complained of a stomachache and headache, which seems to resolve when he gets to school. You have often thought he was pretending to try and get out of school but pleased that he is always better when he gets there.

You have been more forgetful over the past fortnight. You saw your GP who checked you over and took blood tests, but everything was normal and he agreed that you were probably working too hard.

You were feeling quite dizzy and lightheaded today, and had to go out to do the weekly food shop when you collapsed. A passer-by saw the incident and came over to help but you came around within a few moments.

If asked, you live in a small house with a loft conversion. You have your office upstairs and recently bought a gas space heater for the winter months. You have recently had your boiler checked and it was working fine. You possibly have a carbon monoxide meter, somewhere, but you have not seen it for a couple of years. You are not worried about this, as you have checked your boiler. You have a partner who you sometimes stay with over the weekends. You note your symptoms are much better during your time away, but again you put that down to lack of work stress. You do not think you are pregnant.

Mark Scheme – CO poisoning

Task	Achieved	Not-Achieved
Introduction, consent and washing hands		
Takes appropriate history of presenting complaint		
Past medical history including smoking history		
Asks about exacerbating and relieving factors		
Asks if anyone else is unwell at home		
Asks about any new home appliances		
Asks if she has a carbon monoxide detector		
Uses ABCDE approach		
Asks for ABG		
Asks for HbCO on ABG		
Provides 100% Oxygen therapy		
Considers NIV		
Asks for bloods		
Asks for ECG		
Asks about pregnancy status		
Asks for urinalysis		
States that senior help will be required/calls for help		
Knows the difference in CO half life with or without supplemental oxygen		
Has an idea to discuss the need for hyperbaric oxygen		
Says it may be unsafe for the patient and others to be at her home		
Examiner's Global Mark	/5	
Actor / Helper's Global Mark	/5	
Total Station Mark	/30	

Learning Points

- Carbon monoxide levels in the blood can be measured as part of the blood gas analysis. Levels of 30% indicates severe exposure but much lower concentrations do not exclude significant poisoning. The relationship between CO levels and severity of poisoning and clinical outcome is poor. Asymptomatic patients with HbCO below 10% may be discharged.

- Pulse oximetry is unreliable as carboxyhaemoglobin mimics oxyhaemoglobin to give a falsely elevated result. Bespoke carboxyhaemoglobin meters are available and avoid the need for invasive blood tests, a real advantage especially in assessing children.

- 100% Oxygen via a non-rebreathe mask reduces the carbon dioxide half-life from 320 minutes to 80 minutes. Hyperbaric oxygen reduces the half-life further, but the evidence for any long-term benefit is uncertain.

18. Febrile neutropenia

Candidate's Instructions

You are a foundation doctor in the Emergency Department majors area and the triage nurse asks you to see a patient with fever and lethargy immediately as she is worried about them. Please take a full history.

After 6 minutes the examiner will stop you and ask you to summarise back your findings, suggest your differential diagnoses and your initial management plan.

Examiner's Instructions

The candidate is a foundation doctor in the Emergency Department majors area who has been asked to see a patient with fever and lethargy immediately as the triage nurse is worried about them.

The patient is a 52-year-old woman who has recently in the last 2 months been diagnosed with acute leukaemia and has just had their first course of chemotherapy 7 days ago. They started developing a cough with yellowish sputum yesterday and today have felt more unwell with chills. They recorded a temperature 1 hour ago and it was 38.2 C.

The candidate should take a focused history, identify the risk of potential neutropenic sepsis and initiate treatments within the hour.Wherever possible blood cultures should be taken prior to giving antibiotics however this should not delay treatment (including antibiotic administration). Other relevant investigations include blood tests chest x-ray, sputum culture, urine MCS.

Actor's Instructions

You are a 52-year-old woman currently working as a receptionist. You have been recently (in the last 2 months) been diagnosed with acute leukaemia, you have just had your first course of chemotherapy 7 days ago. You started developing a cough with yellowish sputum yesterday and today have felt more unwell with chills. You recorded your temperature 1 hour ago and it was 38.2 C. Your husband was concerned and thought you should go to the ED to get yourself checked. You were fit and well until feeling tired and losing weight in the past 3 months leading to your diagnosis. You never smoked or drank alcohol, and never took any regular medication apart from the occasional paracetamol for headache. You have no medication allergies. You have not left the country in the past year.

You decline pain relief if offered, as you are comfortable sitting in a chair in the triage room.

You should not volunteer information unless asked. The reason you came to the ED is because of the fever and chills. If asked about cough, you have had one with yellowish sputum.

If asked about past medical history you have just started chemotherapy for leukaemia. If asked to clarify the timing of it you then reveal that the first dose was given 7 days ago.

Mark Scheme: Febrile neutropenia

Task	Achieved	Not-Achieved
Introduces self and washes hands		
Confirms patient identity and obtains consent		
Asks about comfort and offers pain relief		
Takes history/communicates in concise manner		
Takes methodical history		
Starts with open question		
Establishes presenting complaint		
Asks about onset and duration of fever		
Asks about severity/grade of fever		
Asks about associated symptoms and cough		
Asks about foreign travel		
Asks about past medical history		
Determines timing of chemotherapy		
Asks medication history including allergies		
Asks about social history including smoking/alcohol		
Differential diagnosis includes febrile neutropenia		
Describes appropriate investigations/management		
Blood cultures in management plan		
States IV antibiotic must be given within 1 hour, not waiting for blood test results		
Specifically mentions need for barrier nursing		
Examiner's Global Mark	/5	
Actor / Helper's Global Mark	/5	
Total Station Mark	/30	

Learning points

- Patients with febrile neutropenia can lack localising features of infection due to a diminished immune response. Neutropenic sepsis also may present without a fever so a low threshold is needed in patients who have had recent chemotherapy.

- These patients can rapidly deteriorate and should be flagged up in the ED triage and immediately assessed. Early investigations and treatment with IV antibiotics should be started within 1 hour of recognition.

- Do not delay giving antibiotics whilst waiting for blood tests to confirm neutropenia. Blood cultures should be taken prior to giving antibiotics but this should not delay giving antibiotics.

19. GORD

Candidate's Instructions

You are the foundation doctor working in the emergency department. A 35-year-old female has been brought into the ED with vomiting and abdominal pain. Currently the patient is haemodynamically stable and has stopped vomiting. The pain has settled with simple analgesia.

You are asked to take a history from this patient by your registrar and then present a summary of the case to them.

After 6 minutes the examiner will stop you and ask you to summarise back your findings, suggest your differential diagnoses and your initial management plan.

Examiner's Instructions

A 35-year-old female has been brought into the emergency department with vomiting and abdominal pain. Currently the patient is haemodynamically stable and has stopped vomiting. The pain has settled with simple analgesia.

The candidate has been asked to take the history from the patient and present the case back to you. Allow the candidate to take a history in the time provided and assess them via the mark scheme below.

Two minutes prior to the end of the OSCE stop the candidate and ask them to repeat a summary of the patient's history back to you.

Actor's Instructions

You are a 35-year-old female who has come into the emergency department with vomiting and upper abdominal pain. You have now stopped vomiting since arrival. A doctor is coming to assess you but you can only give information when asked about it specifically.

Your abdominal pain has been coming and going for 6 months now but got worse today at 7am so you decided to go to the ED. It is at the top and centre of your abdomen near to your chest. It is a burning sensation and sometimes radiates upwards towards your throat. The pain score is around 3/10 usually but today was 7/10 and you vomited twice 30 minutes after waking up. You have not vomited with it previously. The pain seems to come on when you are lying down. You have found that this pain comes and goes every few weeks and tends to be worse when you've been drinking alcohol or had a large or spicy meal. It has improved today with two co-codamol 8/500mg.

You have also noticed you have been belching more lately and sometimes watery liquid comes into the back of your mouth - it tastes horrible! After this has happened you find it painful to swallow but are still able to swallow liquids and solids.

Other than that, your bowel habit has been normal recently. You go once a day with no blood or mucus in stools, or black stools. Your abdomen doesn't feel distended and you are passing wind as usual.

You have no loss of appetite or weight loss and have actually gained 4 stone over the last year. You are not sure why and are seeing your GP for this but think you probably don't have the best diet.

You deny any abnormal vaginal discharge, urinary symptoms (pain on passing urine, frequency), and change in urine colour or yellowing of skin or eyes. You feel it's very unlikely you are pregnant although it isn't impossible. Your LMP was 3 months ago - you are usually fairly irregular due to polycystic ovarian syndrome.

You have not had fever or rigors and don't feel clammy, dizzy or fatigued. You have no other issues such as joint pain, rashes or obvious lumps in neck/axilla/groin.

You have a previous medical history of PCOS and migraine. Your current medications are metformin 500mg BD and Sumatriptan when you have a migraine. You also take the progesterone only pill. You have no known drug allergies. You have no other medical history or surgical history and no known family history of any diseases.

You are unemployed and live with your husband. You don't smoke but enjoy a bottle of vodka at the weekend.

You don't know what has caused this episode but think you need an urgent scan to find out what it is and will be annoyed if you don't get one without good reason.

Mark Scheme - GORD

Task	Achieved	Not Achieved
Introduces self and washes hands.		
Checks patient details and obtains consent		
Builds Rapport with patient		
Elicits detailed history of complaint from the patient.		
Starts with an open question and then moves to closed questions.		
Asks all questions pertinent to GI history.		
Asks pertinent gynaecology history		
Ask about red flags such as weight loss, anorexia, blood in stools, haematemesis, dysphagia		
Elicits important negatives within the history.		
Does a general systemic review for any other symptoms not previously mentioned.		
Asks about previous medical history and surgical history		
Asks about any family history of cancer and also GIT disorders.		
Gets an accurate drug and allergy history.		
Asks about smoking and alcohol and also functional status and job		
Clarifies and summarises the history back to the patient.		
Elicits the patient's ideas, concerns and expectations.		
Summarises the case concisely to the examiner with relevant positive and negative points of the history and possible diagnoses.		
Manages the patient in a caring yet professional manner when upset or worried.		
Able to fluidly take a history and elicit the pertinent symptoms from the patient.		
Forms a good relationship with the patient along the course of the history.		
Examiner's Global Mark	/5	
Actor / Helper's Global Mark	/5	
Total Station Mark	/30	

Learning points:

- The underlying cause of reflux is due to weakness or abnormal relaxation of the lower oesophageal sphincter allowing stomach content to regurgitate back into the oesophagus.

- Risk factors which increase the likelihood of GORD include: Hiatus hernia, Obesity and pregnancy (due to increased intra-abdominal pressure), Smoking, Diabetes or any condition causing gastric stasis, Zollinger Ellison Syndrome (increased gastrin production) and medications such as NSAIDs or prednisolone.

- GORD causes mucosal inflammation of the oesophagus. This can lead to several sequalae, including:

  - Reflux oesophagitis: ulcers and inflammation near the junction of the stomach and oesophagus.

  - Oesophageal strictures - persistent narrowing of the oesophagus caused by inflammation.

  - Barrett's Oesophagus - metaplasia (change of squamous to intestinal columnar epithelium) of the distal Oesophagus. This is a pre-cancerous change and needs regular monitoring.

  - Oesophageal carcinoma.

20. Haematuria

Candidate's Instructions:

A 68-year-old woman presents to the Urgent Care Centre complaining of haematuria. You are the foundation doctor on rotation and are asked to take the initial history and to present back to your supervisor. Plesae take a full history.

After 6 minutes the examiner will stop you and ask you to summarise back your findings, suggest your differential diagnoses and your initial management plan.

Examiner's Instructions:

A 68-year-old woman presents to the Urgent Care Centre complaining of haematuria. The candidate is asked to take the initial history and present it back to the examiner as well as propose a likely diagnosis.

At 6 minutes please ask the candidate to present their findings and diagnosis.

Actor's Instructions

You are a 68-year-old woman who has presented to the Urgent Care Centre today with blood in her urine.

You first noticed the blood last week and a few more times since. You heard an advert on the radio today telling people that if you have blood in your urine you should tell your GP.

Throughout the consultation you appear progressively more anxious. If probed you mention that the radio advert mentioned cancer and that you are very scared.

You describe it as dark red blood mixed in with the urine. You think there may be small clots. There is a bit of blood on the tissue after wiping.

You have not had any pain on passing urine and no pain in the abdomen or loins. If asked, you have noticed that you have been passing urine more frequently. You do not think you have been passing any more or less urine than usual.

You have not noticed any other bleeding or increased bruising.

You have been mostly well in yourself, no recent infections (including urinary infections) and no trauma. You have noticed some increased tiredness however.

Your GP has recently started you on Ramipril for high blood pressure. Other than that you are fit and well, never had any previous surgery, do not have allergies and are not taking any other regular medication. If asked about over the counter medications you volunteer that you occasionally take paracetamol for headaches.

You have smoked 5 cigarettes a day for the past 30 years. You drink alcohol only on special occasions. You have not been travelling abroad for many years. You are now retired but you used to work in a local rubber Wellington boot factory.

Your mother and father both passed away of heart problems in their seventies. You are unaware of any other health problems running in the family.

If asked specifically you can mention the following:

You are pleased as you have lost some of your appetite and about a stone in weight over the past 2 months.

You have not had joint pain, back pain, changes in your vision, changes in your bowel habit, vaginal discharge, shortness of breath or ankle swelling.

You no longer have periods as you went through the menopause 15 years ago.

Mark Scheme: Haematuria

Task	Achieved	Not Achieved
Introduces self, washes hands and checks patient identity		
Opens consultation with use of open questions		
Asks about nature of bleeding		
Asks about associated symptoms including pain and other urinary symptoms		
Asks about recent infections		
Asks about other bleeding and bruising		
Asks about known medical problems		
Asks about history of renal disorders		
Asks about history of cancers		
Asks about previous surgery		
Asks about current medication and recent use of antibiotics		
Asks about: smoking history, alcohol intake and recent travel		
Asks about family history of cancers		
Asks about family history of clotting disorders		
Asks about appetite and weight loss		
Asks about joint pain/swelling		
Asks about change in bowel habit		
Asks about reproductive symptoms- menorrhea and vaginal discharge		
Explores patient's Ideas, Concerns and Expectations		
Correctly identifies high likely of bladder cancer diagnosis		
Examiner's Global Mark	/5	
Actor / Helper's Global Mark	/5	
Total Station Mark	/30	

Learning Points

- Remembering to take a detailed but focused history of other systems can provide valuable clues as to the diagnosis.

- Being familiar with a surgical sieve mnemonic can ensure that you are exploring a comprehensive range of possible diagnoses. In this case you could use VITAMIN.

  V: vascular – or blood related, in this case clotting disorders.

  I: Infection/Inflammatory - Consider severe urinary tract infection or post- infection reactive glomerulonephropathies.

  T: Traumatic - Trauma to the kidneys can present with micro or macroscopic haematuria.

  A: Autoimmune - Renal vasculitis can lead to haematuria and often also present with proteinuria and other systemic symptoms of vasculitis.

  M: Metabolic- Diabetic nephropathy rarely has haematuria but does present with proteinuria.

  I: iatrogenic/idiopathic (and we can include genetic here) - Post renal biopsy, polycystic kidney disease, drug induced (penicillins or sulphonamides).

  N: Neoplastic- Don't just stop and think about cancer but consider where in the body the cancer may be. In this case the timing of haematuria can provide clues - early stream indicates urethral, end stream bladder and continuous more ureter or renal.

- Do not neglect the points you will receive for your communication skills. In such a station taking notice of the patient's nervousness and exploring their Ideas, Concerns and Expectations **(ICE)** can gain you vital marks.

21. Gallstones

Candidate's Instructions

Mrs Smith is a 40-year-old woman who has been referred into the Emergency Department team after seeing her GP today with abdominal pain. Please take a full history from the patient.

After 6 minutes the examiner will stop you and ask you to summarise back your findings, suggest your differential diagnoses and your initial management plan.

Examiner's Instructions

The candidate will take a full history of this patient's abdominal pain. At 6 minutes or if the candidate finishes before this time allow them to present a succinct summary of their findings, offer a differential diagnosis and suggest a management plan.

Actor's Instructions

You are a 40-year-old woman and have come to the GP with some abdominal pain.

The pain started badly two days ago so you booked an emergency appointment at your GP. Looking back, you have had a similar niggling pain for a year or so, but didn't think much of it.

The pain is worse after you have had a fatty meal e.g. fish and chips. The pain is sharp in nature and is in the upper right side of your abdomen. It doesn't move anywhere. It is slightly improved with painkillers (paracetamol and ibuprofen). The pain also makes you feel nauseated.

You have not had fevers or chills. You have not had night sweats or weight loss.

You have noticed a change in your stools: they are lighter in colour and float on the surface of the toilet water.

You have noticed that your urine has become very dark.
Your partner has noticed that your eyes looked a little yellow this morning

You have not been out of the country recently.

You have a long term partner and both of you have clear sexual health screens, you have had no other unprotected sexual intercourse. No unwell contacts.

No regular medications, you have never been into hospital before. You have had no operations. You are a bit concerned as you are overweight, you are trying to improve this and are going to slimming world.

You do not drink alcohol. You do not smoke.

Mark Scheme : Gallstones

Tasks	Achieved	Not Achieved
Washes hands and introduces self		
Confirms patient's name and gains consent		
Asks open ended question about why patient is here today		
Asks about main symptoms site of pain, duration, character, radiation		
Asks for any associated symptoms		
Asks if anything makes it worse or better		
Asks for any change in bowel habit and urination		
Asks if patient has noticed a change in the colouring of skin or their eyes.		
Asks past medical history		
Asks for any medications the patient is taking		
Asks for any family history		
Asks for travel history		
Asks sexual history		
Asks alcohol and drug history		
Asks if pain is worsened by eating fatty foods		
Asks for any weight loss		
Asks for any night sweats		
Provides a good summary of the history		
Differential diagnosis to include gall stones		
Suggests an appropriate management plan e.g. analgesia, investigation with ultrasound		
Examiner's Global Mark	/5	
Actor / Helper's Global Mark	/5	
Total Station Mark	/30	

Learning points

- It is Important to ask about travel and sexual history in any patient with jaundice. There are countries with a high prevalence of hepatitis B. Hepatitis B and C can both be sexually transmitted or through blood borne contact.

- One can have obstructive jaundice for multiple reasons, and it is methodical to separate the causes into painful and painless jaundice. Painless jaundice is more concerning as it is suggestive of a malignancy causing obstruction.

- Main diagnostic imaging for cholelithiasis would be ultrasound, with CT/MRI if concerned about malignancy or pancreatitis.

22. Headache History

Candidate's instructions

You are the foundation doctor working in the emergency department. You pick up the notes for the next patient to be seen and the presenting complaint states 'headache'. The patient is a 24-year-old female called Gaby Howard with no previous ED attendances. Take a full history from the patient and address any concerns she has.

After 6 minutes the examiner will stop you and ask you to summarise back your findings, suggest your differential diagnoses and your initial management plan.

Actor's instructions

You are a 24-year-old professional dancer who has attended the emergency department with a headache.

You have had it for 24 hours and have had to miss work this morning. It came on yesterday morning while you were warming up for a rehearsal and gradually became more painful and hasn't eased up since. You have had a few bad headaches in the past two months (similar in nature and lasting 5-6 hours) but this one has lasted longer and just before it came on you noticed your vision wasn't quite right and your hands felt tingly. Although this resolved within 10 minutes it really worried you.

Site	Right side of your head. No focal area of pain.
Onset	During a morning rehearsal 24 hours ago. Came on gradually, progressed over an hour and then peaked in severity and has stayed at the same intensity since.
Character	Pressure/throbbing sensation
Radiation	None
Associated symptoms	Just before the headache came on you noticed spots in your vision and your hands went tingly - this resolved within a few minutes. You have felt sick since the morning it started but have not vomited. No experience of visual loss, blurred or double vision, zig-zag lines, vertigo, weakness, speech disturbance, loss of consciousness or fits. No unusual smells. No fevers, neck pain or rash.
Timing	Not worse at any particular time of day.
Exacerbating/ Relieving factors	Any activity makes it worse, you feel better if you lay down. Paracetamol seemed to help a little. You haven't tried anything else. No light sensitivity, mild noise sensitivity.
Severity	6/10. You slept OK last night but could not attend work this morning.

You are normally fit and well, you have had an ankle injury for the past 2 months for which you have been taking codeine daily, as you have needed to perform despite the injury. This has been much better over the past week so you have not taken any codeine for several days. You also started taking the contraceptive pill (Microgynon®) four months ago to help ease your periods. Your last menstrual period was 3 weeks ago. Your only family history is your mum's stroke. You live with friends, smoke 7-10 cigarettes/day, drink alcohol 2-3 times per month and take no recreational drugs. No recent foreign travel. You are quite stressed at work but no more than usual, you are expected to perform three times a day and often miss meals and don't hydrate as well as you know you should.

You are concerned that you may be experiencing the early symptoms of a stroke. You know that your mother had a headache and problems with her vision a few days prior to having a stroke, which left her unable to move her right side. She was only 62 when this happened. You expect to have a head scan or that you might need to take aspirin to prevent a stroke - as you know that your mother now takes this to prevent a stroke. If the doctor explains why you do not need a scan and fully addresses your concerns then you are content to proceed with the plan they present.

Examiner's Instructions

The candidate is a foundation doctor in the emergency department. They have been asked to see Gaby, a 24-year-old professional dancer who has attended because of a headache. She has undiagnosed migraines, which have been ongoing for a few months and are related to her menstrual cycle. She has several risk factors for migraine including: female, smoking and use of the combined oral contraceptive pill.

She has also been taking codeine on a near daily basis for an ankle injury. She had become a little dependent on it because she cannot take time off work with the injury. Her ankle has improved and she stopped taking codeine a few days ago, putting her at risk of medication overuse headache.

The candidate is expected to take a full history from the patient, decide upon their top three differential diagnoses and formulate a management plan with the patient. Migraine should be identified as a potential diagnosis, but it does not need to be the candidate's primary diagnosis to obtain full marks. They should formulate a clear and safe management plan that involves a neurological examination including fundoscopy.

The patient is worried because her mother had a stroke, which was preceded by some similar features to her current headache. The candidate should identify the patient's concern and address it directly. There is no indication for a head CT and they need to be able to explain this to the concerned patient.

Stop the candidate with two minutes remaining of the station and ask for their differential diagnoses.

Mark Scheme - Febrile neutropenia

Task	Achieved	Not Achieved
Introduces themselves, seeks consent for consultation and washes hands		
Offers analgesia		
Establishes the patient's main issue (presenting complaint)		
Explores the nature of the headache site, onset, character, radiation, severity		
Establishes the onset, timeframe, associated symptoms, aggravating & relieving factors		
Specifically asks about head injury		
Specifically asks about focal neurology		
Specifically asks about visual symptoms		
Ascertains if there are symptoms of meningitis		
Check for other red flags		
Takes a past medical history		
Takes a drug history		
Takes a family and social history		
Explores the patient's ideas, concerns and expectations		
Establishes a safe and clear management plan		
Checks understanding & invites questions		
Closes the consultation appropriately		
Identifies three reasonable differential diagnoses		
Summarises and signposts during the consultation		
Appropriate language throughout. Avoids medical terminology		
Examiner's Global Mark	/5	
Actor / Helper's Global Mark	/5	
Total Station Mark	/30	

Learning points

- Headaches are a common presenting complaint in the emergency department and these can be very rewarding consultations because most headache diagnoses can be made with a thorough history.

- Headaches have a broad spectrum of underlying causes from the common and benign to the rare and life threatening and therefore need to be treated with a generous dose of suspicion. Some patients will need urgent investigation and treatment whereas others will require nothing more than reassurance, and a solid follow up plan that includes a clear safety net in case things deteriorate.

- You cannot plan for every possible clinical scenario that may arise, but you can have a framework that guides your consultation. This should include appropriate introduction, informal consent, open questions followed by focused questioning, summarising and signposting to ensure accuracy and provide structure to the consultation as well as specifically addressing ideas, concerns and expectations. Give the patient time to talk and be sympathetic and considerate, you will find most consultations flow a lot easier if the patient's agenda is established near the start.

23. Subarachnoid Haemorrhage

Candidate's Instructions

You are the foundation year doctor in the Emergency Department and have been asked to see a 46-year-old woman who has attended with a headache which they are finding difficult to manage. Please take a focused history.

After 6 minutes the examiner will stop you and ask you to summarise back your findings, suggest your differential diagnoses and your initial management plan.

Examiner's Instructions

A 46-year-old female has presented to the emergency department with symptoms consistent with a spontaneous subarachnoid haemorrhage.

The student must take a concise and systematic clinical history before summarizing their findings and stating an initial management plan.

Actor's Instructions

You are a 46-year-old female who was out running when you experienced a sudden onset occipital headache (back of head). You had to stop running immediately as you felt faint and dizzy. It's the worst headache you've ever had and it came on all of a sudden. One minute you were running the next moment you felt this pain in the back of the head almost like you had been hit from behind (describe it in this way only if directly asked). You came straight to the emergency department. The headache is still there and now your neck is feeling stiff.

You have not experienced any vomiting or other symptoms. There are no other neurological signs or symptoms. You are alert and aware of what has happened but are feeling very anxious as this is not normal for you.

Your past medical history include hypertension, for which you take Amlodipine and Ramipril. You get occasional headaches like anyone else but nothing of this magnitude.

You've had no recent trauma and have otherwise been well.

You have you never taken illicit drugs and you drink occasionally.

Mark Scheme

Task	Achieved	Not Achieved
Introduces self, washes hands and confirms name		
Establishes occipital headache and is the worst ever (thunderclap headache)		
SOCRATES of headache		
Asks for triggers – period, cheese, wine, chocolate or stress		
Asks about Neurological deficits – weakness, sensory disturbance, impaired coordination, cognitive symptoms, altered level of consciousness		
Asks about photophobia, neck stiffness, fever and rash		
Asks about visual disturbances (zig zag lights, Red eye and haloes around lights)		
Asks about Nausea and vomiting		
Asks about weight loss, lethargy and night sweats		
Excludes Temporal region tenderness		
Excludes important negatives – trauma, recent illness		
Asks about past medical history (specifically malignancy)		
Asks about drug history (including illicit drug use)		
Asks about family history		
Summarises: States that given the clinical history, primary concern would be a subarachnoid haemorrhage		
Full set of bloods including coagulation screen		
States that this patient will require an urgent CT head		
Lumbar puncture for xanthochromia if CT head negative		
Hourly neurological observations		
Referral to neurosurgery or the closest neurosurgical center		
Examiner's Global Mark	/5	
Actor / Helper's Global Mark	/5	
Total Station Mark	/30	

Learning Points

- There are lots of red flags with headaches that need to be ruled out. Become familiar with these, as headaches are a common presentation in EM. SIGN provides a comprehensive list of red flags if you are unsure of what red flags are.

- Diagnosis of Subarachnoid haemorrhage
  - Non-contrast CT scan will correctly identify 95% of cases
  - Angiography will increase this to 99%
  - Lumbar puncture should be performed after 12 hours in patients with a highly suggestive clinical history. CT scan is negative in 2% of SAHs. Around 3% of patients with a negative CT scan will prove, on lumbar puncture, to have had a SAH.

- Scoring systems used in Subarachnoid haemorrhage
  - Glasgow Coma Scale
  - WFNS (World Federation of Neurosurgeons)
  - Fisher grading – based on CT appearances
  - Ogilvy and Carter – to predict outcome and determine therapy

24. Head Injury (Minor)

Candidate's Instructions

You are a foundation year doctor working in the Emergency Department and have been asked to see this patient by your consultant. A 45-year-old male patient has attended the following an innocuous head injury at home. He currently has a GCS of 15 and walked into the department.

Please take a focused history and advise the patient about your management plan.

After 6 minutes the examiner will stop you and ask you to summarise back your findings, suggest your differential diagnoses and your initial management plan.

Examiner's Instructions

A 45-year-old male patient has attended the Emergency Department following a head injury at home. He currently has a GCS of 15 and walked into the department.

A foundation doctor working in the ED has been asked to take the history and explain the management plan to the patient. If the candidate states that they would like to perform a full neurological examination, state that this is normal, and move them on to explaining a management plan for the patient.

The patient is concerned that there is bleeding in his brain and will request a scan. He becomes annoyed with the junior doctor if told there is no indication for a scan however if relevant guidelines are explained to him then he will be reassured.

Actor's Instructions

You are a 45-year-old man who has attended the Emergency Department following a head injury. You were building a new shed in the garden when you hit the back of your head on a wooden beam.

You have no other injuries and there is no boggy swelling. You did not lose consciousness at the time, however have been feeling unwell, nauseous and dizzy since the injury. If the candidate asks you about vomiting, state that you have not vomited after the accident. You can remember all events leading up to and after the injury and you did not have a seizure. If asked you also mention that your walking and speech has been unchanged since the injury. There hasn't been any clear fluid or blood from either your nose or ears.

You took some painkillers at home as you had a headache but when your wife returned home a few hours later, she was concerned as you looked pale, had a lump at the back of your head and a persistent headache. She told you to attend the ED to get a scan to check for bleeding.

You are previously fit and well and don't take any medication. You have no allergies. You work as a manager on a building site and if prompted by the candidate disclose that you are worried about bleeding in the brain as you have done some reading on the Internet. You would like a quick scan before going home.

If the doctor tells you there is no indication for a CT scan of your head, you become annoyed. However if the candidate explores your concerns and explains the guidelines and indications for a scan then you are reassured. You return to being pleasant if the doctor also provides written head injury advice in the form of an information leaflet and adequate safety netting.

Mark Scheme - Head Injury (Minor)

Task	Achieved	Not Achieved
Introduces self and clarifies patient's identity		
Offers analgesia / checks patient is comfortable		
Uses open questions to begin consultation		
Inquires about mechanism of injury		
Inquires about drops in GCS		
Mentions signs of basal skull fracture		
Mentions open or depressed skull fracture		
Asks about post traumatic seizure		
Loss of consciousness		
Focal neurological deficit		
Vomiting episodes		
Amnesia (30 minutes Retrograde or Antegrade)		
Asks about past medical history, medication history and social history		
Mentions need to perform full neurological examination of patient		
Enquires about patient's ideas, concerns and expectations		
Gives explanation of likely diagnosis to patient i.e. Concussion/minor head injury		
Advises no need for further imaging		
Reassures patient and alludes to NICE head injury guidelines		
Mentions provision of written head injury advice on discharge		
Closes the consultation appropriately with appropriate safety net advice		
Examiner's Global Mark	/5	
Actor / Helper's Global Mark	/5	
Total Station Mark	/30	

Learning points

- Knowing the NICE head injury guidelines is essential and should guide your clinical practice when faced with head injury patients. Utilising evidence based guidelines allows the clinician to use validated decision making to reassure both the patient and the clinical team.

- Try to elicit patient's ideas, concerns and expectations regarding their presentation to the department. Ensuring these are addressed will improve overall patient satisfaction. Communication here is the key to a happy patient.

- Always provide both verbal and written head injury advice upon discharge from the department, appropriate safety-net advice is important.

25. Paracetamol OD

Candidate's instructions

You are the foundation doctor in the Emergency Department. Your next patient, 25-year-old James, has been brought in by his friends. They tell the triage nurse they found him unconscious at home with empty bottles of vodka and paracetamol packets around him. He is now alert but refusing to talk to the triage nurse. Please take a full history.

After 6 minutes the examiner will stop you and ask you to summarise back your findings, suggest your differential diagnoses and your initial management plan.

Examiner's instructions

This station examines the candidate's knowledge of the management of a paracetamol overdose as well as their risk assessment of a patient with self harm and their psychiatric history skills. Establishing a rapport with the patient in the time available is obviously challenging. So, as long as the candidate illustrates that they are making an attempt to put the patient at ease, the patient should open up and give the required information. If the candidate does not demonstrate an empathetic attitude, the patient will shut down and this will become a very difficult station. They can however pick up marks during the discussion at the end with their basic knowledge about a paracetamol overdose.

After 6 minutes stop the candidate and ask them to summarise their findings. They should be able to present in an efficient and succinct manner, establishing that this patient took a paracetamol overdose 6 hours ago, at a possibly toxic level, in what was a high-risk suicide attempt! Their initial management should include baseline blood tests (as outlined in the mark scheme) with a paracetamol level (as it has been more than 4 hours since the overdose). They should be able to explain the need to calculate how much was ingested in mg/kg. Toxicity is unlikely to occur under a dose of 75mg/kg. Knowledge of the mg/kg dose is not expected.

There is normally no need to start NAC without a paracetamol level as long as the result can be obtained and acted on within 8 hours. However treatment should not be delayed if more than 150mg/kg has been ingested. Again, the mg/kg dose is not required, but candidates should be aware that it is reasonable to wait for a paracetamol level (unless a very high dose has been ingested).

Ask them what resources they can use to establish whether or not treatment is required. They should be aware of the paracetamol overdose nomogram and suggest consulting toxbase to guide management. They should know that N-Acetylcysteine (NAC) would be the treatment of choice.

Actor's instructions

You do not want to talk to the doctor. You have been low in mood for about 6 months now. You attempted suicide with the intention of ending your life. You still feel low in mood and you are still having suicidal thoughts. You should initially give one-word answers and make it very clear that you do not want to talk. The candidate should be able to identify this and make an effort to put you at ease. They should ask open questions and give you time to talk. If they are clearly making an attempt to create a rapport you should start to open up and talk to them more.

You have been planning this suicide attempt for a month now. You have researched how much paracetamol to take in order to end your life and have been collecting tablets for a week. You chose last night as the appropriate time as it was your ex-girlfriend's birthday. You broke up 6 months ago and this is when your low mood started. You drank 1 litre of vodka before taking the tablets. You took about half of the tablets you had bought and then vomited and passed out because you were so drunk. Judging from the packets your friends found around you, you estimate that you took around 40 tablets at 8pm, each one containing 500mg of paracetamol. You did not take any other tablets.

You do not use recreational drugs. You had no intention of being discovered and told your friends you were staying at your parents' house. They have been worried about you lately so rang your parents to check, and when they realised you were not there, they rushed to your house and found you. You had left a note to your family and another to your girlfriend explaining why you felt you had to do this. It was very much your intention to end you life. You still feel as though you don't want to live. You feel stupid that you didn't even manage to kill yourself and given the chance you know you'd try again and do it right next time.

You have been feeling hopeless and worthless since you broke up with your girlfriend. You do not see the point in living if you can't be with her. You cannot think of anything to look forward to in the future. You have never been depressed in the past and have never attempted suicide before. You have not been taking care of yourself lately, have been drinking daily, have called in sick to work a number of times and have not really been eating. You have insight into your condition and you know that you are depressed but you have such a low opinion of yourself that you don't feel like it's been important enough to seek help.

You do have a good network of friends and a supportive family but you have not wanted to burden them with your problems so have isolated yourself from them recently. You know they are worried but you feel it will be better for you and them if you were not alive and not around to bring them down. You don't have children.

The candidate may explain to you that you will need to stay in hospital for medical treatment and you will need to talk to the psychiatric team. At this stage you are too apathetic and low in energy to object. You don't want to have to go over the events again but at the moment your response is: 'whatever, I don't care any more.'

Mark Scheme - Paracetamol OD

Task	Achieved	Not Achieved
Introduces self and washes hand		
Is able to encourage the patient to give the history of the overdose attempt.		
Specifically asks about type and time of overdose and the number of pills taken to establish the need for medical treatment.		
Asks about the circumstances of the overdose.		
Asks about the history of the depressive episode. Duration and associated symptoms of depression.		
Asks about previous episodes and suicide attempts		
Asks about alcohol and other substance abuse		
Specifically asks about the intention of the attempt		
Asks about protective factors		
Establishes how the patient is feeling now		
Establishes the patient's willingness to comply with treatment		
Reacts to the patient in a professional, empathic and non judgmental manner		
Is able to summarise findings		
Correctly identifies the high-risk nature of the suicide attempt and knows that this patient should not be permitted to leave the hospital.		
Is aware of the treatment nomogram for a paracetamol overdose and knows that it is based on the time since the overdose and the paracetamol level.		
Knows that over a certain mg/kg dose treatment should not be delayed if the paracetamol level is not available quickly.		
Outlines the baseline investigations including LFTs, paracetamol level, coagulation profile, blood gas for lactate and pH.		
Suggests N-Acetylcysteine as the treatment for the overdose		
Suggests trust guidelines and toxbase as resources to help establish whether treatment is required.		
Knows that a psychiatric referral is required for this patient.		
Examiner's global mark	/5	
Actor's global mark	/5	
Total station mark	/30	

Learning points

- A paracetamol level is only useful if the patient is presenting 4 hours or more since ingesting the paracetamol. Their mg/kg dose of paracetamol should be calculated. Once the paracetamol level is known it should be plotted on the paracetamol overdose nomogram.

- Any evidence of liver damage in the form of newly deranged ALT/AST and clotting also requires treatment.

- Have an idea how you are planning on asking the questions. These questions are quite clearly of a sensitive nature which may cause you to tumble over your words. For example; If you want to know if someone is suicidal, try an open question such as, 'how do you feel now?' and then 'do you still feel like you want to end your life?' as supposed to something very blunt like 'do you want to die?'.

26. Pancreatitis

Candidate's Instructions:

You are the foundation doctor in the Emergency Department majors area. A 54-year-old is brought to the ED by ambulance after developing a sudden onset of severe epigastric abdominal pain radiating through to her back for the last 24 hours. She has now developed vomiting and a temperature. Please take a full history from the patient.

After 6 minutes the examiner will stop you and ask you to summarise back your findings, suggest your differential diagnoses and your initial management plan.

Examiner's Instructions:

A 54-year-old lady who has been brought in with a 24 hour history of epigastric pain radiating to her back and has now developed vomiting and a temperature.

The candidate should take a clear and concise history regarding the presentation but should also ask about:

PMH: Gastroesophageal reflux

DH: Takes prednisolone regularly for her Polymyalgia rheumatica (PMR) and

SH: Where she consumes a bottle of wine an evening with dinner and may have a gin and tonic or 2 at lunchtime.

At 6 minutes, please stop the candidate at whatever point they are at in the history and ask them to summarise their findings and ask what differentials they can decipher from their history.

Actor's Instructions:

You are a 54-year-old housewife who suddenly developed severe epigastric pain 24 hours ago. You find the pain excruciating and groan intermittently throughout the history. You thought it was reflux so took two omeprazole tablets but it made no difference. You've now had continuous vomiting since you woke up this morning and feel very unwell.

The pain is located in the middle just below chest level and goes into the back. It's constant dull ache with intermittent sharp episodes. You've never had anything like this before. Not aggravate or relieved by anything.

You've had a small amount of diarrhoea but it's more the vomiting you're worried about.

You have a past medical history of Reflux, hypertension and Polymyalgia rheumatica (PMR). When asked about medications you reply 'Oh nothing dear...well, apart from my omeprazole. Oh and the steroids I take for my PMR. Starts with a P I think...'. You do not have any drug allergies.

You are a Non-smoker and Live with your husband. When asked about alcohol you respond with "a tipple now and again". if pressed for how much per day, "well, a bottle of red in the evening with dinner and maybe a G&T or 2 and some prosecco with the girls when we go out for lunch". You become quite insulted and argumentative if it's insinuated that you're an alcoholic and argue that it must be something else that has caused your symptoms.

Mark Scheme: Pancreatitis

Task	Achieved	Not-Achieved
Introduces self and washes hands		
Checks patient identity and obtains consent		
Asks open question initially		
Use of verbal and non-verbal cues		
Methodical approach to history – SOCRATES		
Asks about gallstones		
Enquires about history of trauma		
Asks about surgical procedures in particular ERCP		
Asks about weight loss, change in bowel habit		
Can ask about any of the less common causes of pancreatitis		
Rules out other similar pathologies e.g reflux, AAA		
Elicits history from parent in a concise manner		
Asks about past medical history		
Asks about drug history & allergies		
Asks about social history		
When evasive re: alcohol consumption, asks for specifics		
Checks units of alcohol consumed per day		
Non-judgemental discussion		
Ideas, Concerns and expectations		
Summarises consultation & actions from here on		
Examiner's Global Mark	/5	
Actor / Helper's Global Mark	/5	
Total Station Mark	/30	

Learning Points

- Pancreatitis is most commonly caused by gallstone or excess alcohol. However tempting to enquire from the patient, the infamous 'scorpion bite' differential diagnosis is unlikely to be the underlying aetiology.

- Good history taking, particularly of the past medical history and social history is essential here. The use of steroids for her PMR as well as her high levels of alcohol would be indicative risk factors for pancreatitis.

- In epigastric pain radiating to the back, ALWAYS exclude aortic pathology especially in patients in their 50s and above. When stratifying pancreatitis the Glasgow Score is still used with three or more of the following indicating severe pancreatitis:

  - Age >55 years
  - WBC >15 x 109/L
  - Urea >16 mmol/L
  - Glucose >10 mmol/L
  - pO2 <8 kPa (60 mm Hg)
  - Albumin <32 g/L
  - Calcium <2 mmol/L
  - LDH >600 units/L
  - AST/ALT >200 units

27. Back Pain History Taking

Candidate's Instructions

You are the foundation year doctor in the Emergency Department in the majors area. A 65-year-old man has been referred in via the GP with a 6-week history of worsening back pain. please take a full history.

After 6 minutes the examiner will stop you and ask you to summarise back your findings, suggest your differential diagnoses and your initial management plan.

Examiner's Instructions

The candidate is a foundation year doctor in the Emergency Department in the majors area who has been asked to see and take a full history from a 65-year-old man referred in via the GP with a 6-week history of worsening back pain.

After 6 minutes, please stop the candidate and ask them:

Which condition are they worried about, and which investigation(s) would they like to order?

Which blood tests would be helpful to further investigate causes of back pain?

Which bedside tests would they like, and any in particular if the patient was a younger female?

If the patient presented with associated incontinence, what should they be worried about and what would be the next step?

Actor's Instructions

You are a 68-year-old man who has been suffering with back pain for 6 weeks.

The pain started slowly, and has been getting progressively worse. There is no specific trigger that has set this pain off but you have put it down to doing extra gardening while the weather has been better. You describe it as an ache that travels into your groin on both sides, sometimes going into your testes. You have not had any weakness or altered sensations in the legs such as pins and needles. Nothing seems to make the pain worse, but paracetamol has helped which you are taking more regularly. You have had back pain in the past, but this was usually following heavy lifting and the episodes all resolved within a week.

Aside from the pain, you have been well in yourself and have not had a cold or flu in years. You eat well and have put on some weight now that the summer is over. Your bowel habit has been regular for as long as you can remember. You have no problems passing water since your prostate surgery 5 years ago.

You have a past medical history of BPH (benign prostatic hyperplasia).

You have high blood pressure and raised cholesterol but do not take any medications for these because of your intolerance of the side effects.

You do not smoke but enjoy a few glasses of wine a day.

You decided to see the doctor as the pain has been getting worse and you are struggling to sleep and do your daily activities. More recently you have been unable to tend the garden. You also are not sure why you have not recovered in 6 weeks. You are worried about cancer because you had prostate problems in the past and one of your friends had prostate cancer that spread to his spine.

Mark Scheme : Back pain

Task	Achieved	Not-Achieved
Introduction and consent		
History of presenting complaint		
Asks appropriate questions about current back pain episode		
Asks about any previous episodes of back pain		
Determines if there are any exacerbating or relieving factors		
Asks about associated fever		
Asks about pins and needles paraesthesia or weakness in legs		
Asks about altered sensation in the bottom, between anus and genitalia		
Asks about bladder dysfunction		
Asks about faecal incontinence		
Asks about drug history, specifically analgesia and long term steroids		
Asks about past medical history		
Asks about impairment to work and lifestyle		
Asks about blood in urine if male, LMP if female		
Determines if there has been any unexpected weight loss		
Elicits patients' ideas, concerns and expectations regarding episode of back pain		
Asks for urine dip and BHCG (if female)		
Asks for blood tests including amylase and bone profile		
Asks for bedside ultrasound scan, or any examination to look at abdominal aortic aneurysm.		
Knows to ask for specialist referral/ imaging if any symptoms of cauda equina syndrome are present		
Examiner's Global Mark	/5	
Actor / Helper's Global Mark	/5	
Total Station Mark	/30	

Learning points

- In the emergency department important it is important to rule out life threatening conditions such as an abdominal aortic aneurysm. These can present very non-specifically and they can be easily missed. In any older patient with back pain, check the abdominal aorta!

- Another important cause of back pain to be ruled out is cauda equina syndrome. Prompt investigation and management is required as the longer the nerve is compressed or damaged the worse the function and ultimately the recovery will be. MRI would be

- Red Flags, I.e. criteria for further investigation, include:
    - Extremes of age
    - Non mechanical pain
    - Saddle anaesthesia
    - Bladder or bowel dysfunction
    - Weakness in the lower limbs
    - Weight loss
    - Fever
    - Thoracic pain

28. Pericarditis

Candidate's Instructions

You are the foundation doctor in the Emergency Department in the majors area. Your next patient is a 24-year-old man with chest pain. He has been here an hour waiting to be seen. Please take a history and tell him the likely diagnosis and your management plan.

After 6 minutes the examiner will stop you and ask you to summarise back your findings, suggest your differential diagnoses and your initial management plan

Examiner's Instructions

The candidate is a foundation doctor in the Emergency Department in the majors area who has been asked to see a 24-year-old man with chest pain and take a full history and decide upon the likely differential diagnoses and the initial management plan.

After 6 minutes stop the candidate and ask them to summarise back their findings, suggest differential diagnoses and the initial management plan.

Actor's Instructions

You are a 24-year-old university student studying history. You suddenly felt a sharp pain in the middle of your chest this afternoon at around 2pm today while sitting in the library revising for an exam.

It felt like someone was stabbing you in the chest. The pain was worse when you took a breath in or moved and felt better when you leaned or sat forward. At worst the pain can be described as the worst pain you have ever felt. You went home and lay down in bed but felt this made the pain worse. You also feel a dull pain in your left shoulder, which comes and goes.

Your housemate felt you looked uncomfortable and thought you should go to the Emergency Department. Before you left for the ED you had a dose of Ibuprofen, now the pain is less than half as bad as it was. You are normally well but have felt generally flu-like over the past day, you have no other past medical history.

You don't smoke and you drink an average of 4 pints of lager over the week with friends. You don't take any medication and have no allergies. Your father has a history of high blood pressure and takes medication for it.

If asked, you decline pain relief as you feel the pain is tolerable after the ibuprofen. When the candidate gives you their diagnosis you get slightly anxious and ask 'is it serious doctor?'

Mark Scheme: Pericarditis

Task	Achieved	Not Achieved
Introduces self and washes hand		
Confirms patient identity and gains consent		
Asks about comfort and offers pain relief		
Takes history/communicates in concise manner		
Takes methodical history		
Checks for preceding illness eg viral illness		
Asks about site		
Asks about onset		
Asks about character		
Asks about radiation		
Asks about associated symptoms		
Asks about timing/duration		
Asks about exacerbating/relieving factors		
Asks about severity		
Asks about past medical history/risk factors		
Asks about medication/allergies		
Asks about Social history including smoking/alcohol		
Describes likely diagnosis to patient		
Offers Reassurance		
Describes appropriate management plan		
Examiner's Global Mark	/5	
Actor / Helper's Global Mark	/5	
Total Station Mark	/30	

Learning points

- The most common cause of acute pericarditis in young people is viral in origin. Viral pericarditis is usually benign and self-limiting; treatment is symptomatic with NSAIDS and bed rest.

- Investigations include, ECG (may be diagnostic), chest x-ray, troponin/cardiac enzymes may also be raised if there is associated myocarditis.

- Concerning features include raised fever (>38 C), signs of pericardial effusion, myocarditis, history of immunosuppression, autoimmune disease, recent MI, or recent trauma. These patients may need admission for urgent echo and monitoring.

29. PR BLEED

Candidate's Instructions:

You are the foundation doctor in the Emergency Department in the majors area. You have been asked by your consultant to see a 54-year-old man has been brought to the ED with a PR bleed. Currently the man is haemodynamically stable but reports feeling nauseous and seeing fresh red blood coming from the back passage. Please take a full history.

After 6 minutes the examiner will stop you and ask you to summarise back your findings, suggest your differential diagnoses and your initial management plan.

Examiner's Instructions:

A 54-year-old man has been brought to the Emergency department with a PR bleed. Currently the man is haemodynamically stable but reports feeling nauseated and seeing fresh red blood coming from the back passage.

The foundation doctor in the emergency medicine team has been asked to take the initial history and also ascertain if there are any red flags present in this patient in relation to the PR bleed. Allow the candidate to take a history in the time provided and carefully elicit if they ask about red flag symptoms and signs.

After 6 minutes stop the candidate and ask them to present back their findings, the differential diagnoses and list the signs and symptoms of red flags in a patient with a PR bleed.

Actor's Instructions:

You are a 54-year-old man who has presented to the emergency department with fresh red blood coming from the back passage/bottom. You find it hard to quantify the amount of blood. It is mixed in with stool and seen on the toilet paper. Your bowel habit has been slightly constipated recently. You have been going less often and have noticed in the last month that your stool is darker, almost black in colour! This is the first time you have noticed any blood. You have not noticed any mucous in the stool. You deny having any abdominal pain.

You have not vomited but feel nauseated and have been eating and drinking less generally for the last 2 months as you have been less hungry than usual. You have lost a stone over this time but it was unintentional.

You have not had fever or rigors but currently feel clammy.

You deny any urinary symptoms, change in urine colour or yellowing of skin or eyes. You are passing flatus as usual and do not have abdominal distension. You haven't been feeling dizzy, tired or short of breath recently.

You have no other issues such as joint pain, rashes, or obvious lumps in neck/axilla/groin.

You have a previous medical history of a mild heart attack two years ago, which is medically treated with daily aspirin, bisoprolol and simvastatin. You have no known drug allergies. You have no other medical history but did have an operation on your haemorrhoids four years ago.

Your mum died from ovarian cancer, aged 80 and your Dad is still alive and well. Your paternal grandmother died of a heart attack. There are no other medical issues you are aware of in your family.

You currently live with your wife and are fully independent. You do not smoke but enjoy a drink regularly - you drink 2 pints of Guinness a night and also drink around about a bottle of whiskey each weekend. You work as a pub landlord.

You have no idea what has caused this episode but are very concerned it could be cancer and keep asking if the doctor thinks that is what it is.

Mark Scheme : PR bleed

Task	Achieved	Not Achieved
introduces self and washes hands		
Clarifies who they are speaking to and gains consent		
Starts with an open question and then moves to closed questions.		
Clarifies that this Is not haematuria or vaginal bleeding		
Frequency and amount		
Asks if Blood is mixed in with the stool, around the stool, on the pan, or on the tissue paper		
Establishes character: fresh blood, melaena, clots, muscus, smell		
Asks about exacerbating or alleviating factors (relieved by defecation, dietary or foreign body history)		
Ask about associated symptom (dragging sensation, tenesmus, itching and pain)		
Elicits if important red flag symptoms are present (haemetemesis, weight loss, loss of appetite and change in bowel habit)		
Asks about bleeding from elsewhere		
Does a general systemic review for any other symptoms not previously mentioned.		
Asks about previous medical history		
Asks about any surgical history		
Asks about any family history of cancer and GI disorders (e.g. angiodysplasia or IBD)		
Gets an accurate drug and allergy history (specifically NSAIDS or anticoagulants)		
Asks about job, smoking and alcohol.		
Elicits the patient's ideas, concerns and expectations.		
Manages the patient in a caring yet professional manner when upset or worried.		
Forms a good relationship with the patient along the course of the history.		
Examiner's Global Mark	/5	
Actor / Helper's Global Mark	/5	
Total Station Mark	/30	

Learning points:

- GI bleeding can originate anywhere from the mouth to the anus and can be overt or occult. How this presents depends on the location and rate of bleeding.

- Red flags of PR bleed include: Weight loss, altered blood PR, change in bowel habit, abdominal pain, mucus passed PR and anorexia.

- If the patient is initially haemodynamically unstable the first action must be to do an A to E assessment with appropriate interventions along the way - two large bore cannula, bloods, venous blood gas and Group and Save. Always call for help.

30. Renal Stones

Candidate's Instructions

You are the foundation doctor in the Emergency Department in the majors area. A 30-year-old man self-presents to ED with severe right sided loin pain.
Please take a full history.

After 6 minutes the examiner will stop you and ask you to summarise back your findings, suggest your differential diagnoses and your initial management plan.

Examiner's Instructions

A 30-year-old man self-presents to ED with severe right sided loin pain.

The candidate has been asked to take a history and formulate a management plan.

After 6 minutes please bring the consultation to a close and ask the candidate to present their history and management plan.

If not offered ask the candidate directly about:

- Initial treatment

- Investigations required to confirm diagnosis and exclude complications

- Follow up plans

Actor's Instructions

You are a 30-year-old man who has come to the ED with a 12 hour long episode of worsening right sided back and abdominal pain, you point and hold your right side just below your ribs. During the consultation you are obviously in pain, cannot sit still and cannot get comfortable.

The pain is severe and gripping in nature, coming in waves. It started slowly but progressed rapidly. It moves all the way down to your groin. You feel sick and have vomited once.

If asked specifically, you have noticed:

- An increased frequency, no blood and no pain on passing urine
- no change in bowel habit
- no fever
- no other symptoms

During the consultation you frequently make comments about how much pain you are in and that you would like it to stop.

You are otherwise fit and well, on no regular medications. You do not smoke or drink. You are an avid gym goer and drink regular protein shakes. You remember your dad being hospitalised when you were younger for kidney problems.

Mark Scheme: Renal Stones

Task:	Achieved	Not Achieved
Introduces self, washes hands and checks patient identity		
Opens consultation with use of open questions		
Explores pain history in a systematic manner		
Asks about haematuria		
Explores urinary symptoms		
Asks specifically about previous renal stones		
Explores past medical and surgical history		
Takes a thorough drug history including over the counter and illicit drugs		
Asks about smoking and alcohol history		
Asks about family of renal stones		
Explores a brief system's enquiry		
Explores patient's Ideas, Concerns and Expectations		
Recognizes need for analgesia and reassures patient		
Correctly identifies diagnosis of renal colic		
Asks for a urine dip and justifies to check for microscopic haematuria		
Asks for an FBC and CRP and justifies to check for signs of infection		
Asks for U&Es and justifies to check for acute kidney injury		
Asks for CT KUB and justifies to check for renal stones and urinary obstruction		
States would give Per Rectum diclofenac as first line analgesia		
States next step would require urology inpatient or outpatient review depending on CT scan result and renal function		
Examiner's Global Mark	/5	
Actor / Helper's Global Mark	/5	
Total Station Mark	/30	

Learning Points

- Have a systematic approach to taking a pain history, such as SOCRATES. This will show the examiner that you can take an organized history. It is also vital clinically to get all the information from the patient. Every aspect of pain is a clue to the diagnosis.

- Be specific when providing a management plan in an OSCE. Don't just state the test you would order but add what you are looking for.

- When presenting a history to a senior or colleague having a systematic approach can help you remain concise and still report all the relevant information. SBAR is a commonly used acronym for this

    - The **Situation** is the Presenting problem and suspected likely diagnosis (or main medical problem)

    - The **Background** contains 2 or 3 main facts from the history highlighting the suspected diagnosis and 1 or 2 important negatives that exclude other important differentials. Go on to explain **Assessment** findings.

    - **Recommendation** can be when you outline your management plan or conclude by saying that you would now do a focused examination of the patient.

31. Syncope

Candidate's Instructions

You are the foundation doctor in the Emergency Department in the majors area and have been asked to see a 25-year-old man who has collapsed today. Please take a full history.

After 6 minutes the examiner will stop you and ask you to summarise back your findings, suggest your differential diagnoses and your initial management plan.

Examiner's Instructions

The candidate is a foundation doctor in the Emergency Department in the majors area who has been asked to see a 25-year-old man who has presented after a collapse and take a full history and decide upon the likely differential diagnoses and the initial management plan.

Actor's instructions

You are a 25-year-old man who has presented to your local hospital having had a collapse.

You had just been at the gym and were sat at the bus stop on your way home, you stood up as the bus was approaching and started to feel light headed. Then you noticed your vision going darker and felt that you felt you were spinning. The next thing you knew the man sat next to you at the bus stop was asking if you were ok, and you were on the ground. He called the ambulance.

The man told you that you passed out and did not hit your head. You did not lose control of your bladder or Bowels. You did not bite your tongue. The man looking after you told the paramedics that it didn't look like you had a seizure. You were out for no more than 30 seconds. You have had this once or twice in the past and just put it down to fainting.

You have been feeling well recently but had forgotten to take your water bottle to the gym this morning and pushed yourself a little harder than normal. You are now feeling well and have not had chest pain.

You are otherwise fit and well. You take no regular medications. You have no allergies. You have no significant illness running in your family, no one has any heart problems or epilepsy. You have not been abroad recently. You have occasional alcohol binges "big nights out". You occasionally take MDMA but haven't in the last 3 months.

Mark Scheme

Task	Achieved	Not achieved
Washes hands, Introduces self to patient and confirms identity		
Begins with open ended questions		
Asks about aura/indications		
Asks about what patient was doing preceding the collapse		
Asks about preceding chest pain, dizziness, headache		
Asks if there was any head trauma		
Asks if the collapse was witnessed and what was the account		
Asks questions about a possible seizure, loss of bladder or bowel control, tongue biting		
Asks about conscious level after collapse, was there a period of unresponsiveness (Post-Ictal)		
Asks about past medical history and history of syncope		
Ask after symptoms of meningitis		
Ask about symptoms of malignancy		
Asks drug history including allergies and recreational drugs		
Asks family history- epilepsy, heart valve or heart rhythm problems		
Asks about occupation		
Summarises findings		
Differential diagnosis: vasovagal syncope, arrhythmia, epilepsy		
Investigations: ecg, blood gas,		
Asks for blood sugar level		
Management plan can go home if all tests normal		
Examiners Global Mark	/5	
Patient's Global Mark	/5	
Total station Mark	/30	

Learning points

- Collapse is a very common presentation with a mixture of benign and sinister causes. Have a list of the sinister causes and how to rule them out. E.g. cardiac arrhythmia, check an ECG for conduction abnormalities.

- Categorise collapse into main aetiologies e.g. cardiac valve problems, conduction problems, Neuro: epilepsy, Cardiovascular: vasovagal, micturition syncope, Endocrine: hypoglycaemia. Coareful histroy taking is required and enquiry about the events before, during and after the episode will go a long way in narrowing down your differential diagnoses.

- Collapse in the elderly patients should have infection ruled out, anticoagulation status checked and skeletal injuries considered and excluded, especially the potential for pelvic and neck of femur fractures.

32. Respiratory Examination

Candidate's instructions

You are the foundation doctor in the Emergency Department in the majors area.

A 66-year-old lady has presented to the ED because she has been feeling unwell since getting back from holiday in Australia a week ago. She has had a chesty cough for a few days and awoke this morning shaking and unable to get warm, she is also feeling a bit breathless. She has no history of lung disease or smoking. She is normally fit and well and was swimming daily in the hot springs in Australia while away.

Perform a respiratory examination on this patient and present your findings to the examiner. Outline any bedside investigations that should be performed and how you will manage this patient in the ED.

Examiner's Instructions

The candidate has been asked to perform a respiratory examination on the patient who has presented with symptoms of pneumonia shortly after returning from a holiday in Australia. The candidate should perform a full respiratory examination and present their findings. The examination should be conducted in a methodical manner and with minimal discomfort to the patient, it is therefore preferable to examine the anterior chest all at once and the back all at once, the custom of inspection, palpation, percussion and auscultation should be followed each time.

To extend their initial assessment the candidate should be able to identify at least three bedside tests, accept pulse oximetry, arterial blood gas, sputum sample, blood (specifically inflammatory markers or cultures) and urinary antigen tests. Also award marks for chest x-ray. This lady has symptoms of moderate severity and it would be appropriate to prescribe antibiotics, supportive treatment, symptom control and admit her to hospital.

Stop the candidate 6 minutes into the station and ask, if not already stated, what their primary diagnosis would be at this stage. Ask them to state three findings on examination of the chest that they could expect to find in a patient with pneumonia. Ask if there is an objective scoring system, which can be used to determine the severity of the pneumonia. CRB-65 (accept CURB-65).

Actor's instructions

You are a 66-year-old female who has come to the emergency department as you have been feeling unwell for the past week and have not been able to see your GP.

You returned from visiting your children in Australia just over a week ago and felt unwell the day after your return. You have been coughing for days, more recently bringing up thick green sputum. You have been off your food and have had a few bouts of loose stool. In the past 24 hours you have felt short of breath and this morning you awoke feeling very cold and unable to get warm - you were shivering continuously and so decided to seek emergency care.

The candidate will perform an examination of your chest. You feel breathless and have an increased breathing rate. You don't have any pain.

Mark Scheme : Respiratory examination

Task	Achieved	Not achieved
Introduces themselves and washes hands		
Consents patient and confirms identity		
Asks if the patient has pain & offers analgesia if appropriate		
Positions at 45º and exposes appropriately		
General inspection. Respiratory rate.		
Hands - tobacco staining, tremor, flap, stigmata of disease. Pulse.		
Face - eyes and mouth. Cyanosis, ptosis, conjunctival pallor		
Neck - JVP, tracheal position and lymphadenopathy		
Palpation - chest expansion		
Percussion - clavicles, anterior and posterior		
Auscultation - anterior and posterior		
Checks for either vocal resonance or tactile vocal fremitus		
Pedal and sacral oedema		
Performs examination in a considerate way, maintaining communication and safeguarding patient decency throughout.		
Performed in a systematic and sensible order. Compares the left and right sides.		
Presents their finding in a systematic and clear way		
Identifies the need for vital signs and can name three bedside tests		
Identifies pneumonia as a likely diagnosis		
Formulates an appropriate management plan		
Able to name two clinical findings consistent with pneumonia. Aware of CRB-65/CURB-65 assessment.		
Examiner's Global Mark	/5	
Actor / Helper's Global Mark	/5	
Total Station Mark	/30	

Learning points

- A rehearsed and methodical examination of the respiratory system is a basic clinical skill and you should aim to be comfortable performing this examination. A systematic approach looks professional, helps you to remember all areas to be covered and ensures you aren't moving the patient around unnecessarily.

- CURB 65 is a clinical prediction rule. Each criteria is valued with a point. Points are linked to a 30-day mortality and are used for deciding how to treat the patient. They are marked as follows:

  - Confusion of new onset (defined as an AMTS of 8 or less),
  - Blood Urea nitrogen greater than 7mmol/l (19 mg/dL)
  - Respiratory rate of 30 breaths per minute or greater
  - Blood pressure less than 90 mmHg systolic or diastolic blood pressure below 60mmHg
  - Age 65 or older

- Although ideal, it is not essential to detect all of the clinical signs present in an OSCE examination. It is more important to show that you can perform the examination thoroughly, maintain a professional and polite approach and to show that you are aware of the necessary next steps to ensure that the patient is managed safely.

References

Lim et al. BTS guidelines for the management of community acquired pneumonia in adults:update 2009. A quick reference guide. Thorax 2009.

33. - Cardiovascular examination

Candidate's Instructions

You are the foundation doctor in the Emergency Department in the majors area.

A 69-year-old female patient has been brought into the Emergency Department by ambulance after collapsing outside a shopping centre.

Please examine her cardiovascular system. After 6 minutes the examiner will stop you and ask you to summarise back your findings.

Examiner's Instructions

A 69-year-old female patient has been brought into the Emergency Department by ambulance after collapsing outside a shopping centre. The candidate has been instructed to examine the patient's cardiovascular system.

With two minutes remaining stop them and ask them to describe their examination findings. Do not prompt the candidate in any other way.

Actor's Instructions

You are a 69-year-old woman who has been brought to the Emergency Department by ambulance after collapsing outside your local shopping centre. Please allow the candidate to examine your cardiovascular system.

If the candidate asks, you are not in any discomfort however please make it clear if they cause you any pain.

Mark Scheme: Cardiovascular examination

Task	Achieved	Not achieved
Introduces self and washes hands		
Consents Patient and Checks identity		
Checks patient is comfortable and obtains verbal consent		
Exposes patient adequately and positions patient lying at 45 degree angle		
Performs general inspection from the end of the bed		
Inspects hands - peripheral cyanosis, temperature, nicotine staining, clubbing, signs of infective endocarditis		
Palpates radial pulse (rate, volume, character – slow rising)		
Mentions checking blood pressure		
Assesses Jugular Venous Pressure (JVP) +/- hepatojugular reflux		
Inspects face – corneal arcus, central cyanosis, conjunctival pallor, malar flush		
Palpate carotid artery (volume, character)		
Inspects the precordium – no visible scars		
Palpates for heaves, thrills and apex beat		
Auscultates in correct regions - apex, pulmonary, aortic, tricuspid, mitral		
Performs manoeuvre to accentuate murmur - sits patient forwards and listens with diaphragm in expiration		
Auscultates for radiation of murmur into carotid		
Auscultates lung bases, checks for sacral and ankle oedema		
Thanks patient, offers help in redressing/covering		
Demonstrates systematic approach		
Correctly summarises findings – ejection systolic murmur loudest in aortic region, radiates to carotids		
Examiner's Global Mark	/5	
Actor / Helper's Global Mark	/5	
Total Station Mark	/30	

Learning points

*   When approaching examination stations in the OSCE, always take the time to introduce yourself to the patient and ask them if they are in pain. Being kind and courteous throughout will ensure you pick up the allocated global marks.

*   Clinical features specific to aortic stenosis include: a slow rising pulse, narrow pulse pressure, an ejection systolic murmur heard loudest in the aortic region with radiation into the carotids. There may or may not be signs of heart failure.

*   The correct regions for auscultation are as follows:
    *   Apex – 5th intercostal space, anterior-mid axillary line
    *   Pulmonary – left sternal edge, 2nd-4th intercostal space
    *   Aortic – right sternal edge, 2nd-4th intercostal space
    *   Tricuspid – left sternal edge, 4th-6th intercostal space
    *   Mitral – mid-clavicular line, 4th-6th intercostal space

34. Abdominal examination

Candidate's Instructions

You are the foundation doctor in the Emergency Department in the majors area.

You are asked to see Kieran, a 17-year-old boy who presented to the emergency department with a 2-day history or worsening abdominal pain. He feels nauseous, has a fever and reports 1 episode of loose stools.

Please perform an abdominal examination. After 6 minutes the examiner will stop you and ask you to summarise back your findings and the likely diagnosis.

Examiner's Instructions

Observe this student performing an abdominal examination on a patient with suspected acute appendicitis. After they have finished, they must first summarise their findings before stating the most likely diagnosis and initial management plan.

Actor's Instructions

Your name is Kieran, a 17-year-old student who has had worsening pain in his abdomen for the past 2 days.

The student will perform an examination of your abdomen, but may also look at your hands and face. You have pain in the right lower abdomen, which is very sensitive when touched. Specifically it's a few inches below and across (towards the hip) from your belly button. When your abdomen is felt elsewhere, you also feel pain in your right lower abdomen.

Mark Scheme : Abdominal examination

Task	Achieved	Not Achieved
Introduces self and washes hands		
Confirms patients identity and consents patient		
Positions patient flat, ensures privacy		
Inspection from end of bed: General appearance, high BMI or cachexic, jaundiced, comfortable or in pain		
Inspects the hands: clubbing, leukonychia, koilonychias, palmer erythema, liver flap, pulse		
Inspects the Face: pale conjunctiva in anaemia, yellow sclera in jaundice, mouth for angular stomatitis, dentition, tongue for cyanosis,		
Inspects neck for Virchow's node		
Inspects chest for spider naevi, gynaecomastia		
Inspects abdomen: Distension, abnormal masses, scars from previous surgery		
Palpation of abdomen – nine quadrants, superficially then deep		
Establishes right iliac fossa tenderness		
Checks for peritonism		
Checks for organomegaly of liver and spleen		
Palpates for AAA – expansile and pulsatile mass		
Ballots both kidneys		
Percusses for liver, spleen and bladder		
Auscultates for bowel sounds and aortic renal bruits		
Offers to perform special tests: Rovsing's and Murphy's		
States to complete examination, they would also like to examine external genitalia, hernia orifices, digital rectal examination, urine dip and bedside observations		
Summarises the history and examination consistent with a diagnosis of acute appendicitis		
Examiner's Global Mark	/5	
Actor / Helper's Global Mark	/5	
Total Station Mark	/30	

Learning Points

- Acute appendicitis classically presents with nausea, vomiting, central abdominal pain which migrates to the right iliac fossa and low grade fevers. Examination findings include tenderness and guarding in right iliac fossa (over Mcburneys point), Rovsing's sign, occasionally a mass may be palpable where an appendix abscess has formed.

- Rovsing's Sign- If palpation of the left lower quadrant of the abdomen increases the pain felt in the right lower quadrant, the patient is said to have a positive Rovsing's sign and may have appendicitis.

- Alvarado score (1) for acute appendicitis – a useful diagnostic 'rule out' score. The score is well calibrated in men, inconsistent in children and over-predicts the probability of appendicitis in women. (2)

Use acronym **'MANTRELS'** as memory aid...

Criteria	Yes	No
Abdominal pain which **M**igrates to RIF	1 point	O points
Anorexia (Loss of appetite)	1 point	O points
Nausea and vomiting	1 point	O points
Tenderness in right lower quadrant/RIF	2 point	O points
Rebound tenderness	1 point	O points
Elevated temperature (>37.3C)	1 point	O points
Leukocytosis (WCC > 10)	2 points	O points
Shift of white cells to the left (i.e. neutrophillia)	1 point	O points

Total score:

< 4 - 96% probability diagnosis is not appendicitis

4 <= Score < 7 - Consider imaging (CT/USS)

>7 - Consider surgery (58-88% chance of positive appendicitis)

References:
Alvarado, A (May 1986). "A practical score for the early diagnosis of acute appendicitis.". Annals of Emergency Medicine. 15 (5): 557–64. doi:10.1016/S0196-0644(86)80993-3
Ohle et al.: The Alvarado score for predicting acute appendicitis: a systematic review. BMC Medicine 2011 9:139

35. Cranial Nerve examination

Candidate's instructions

You are the foundation doctor in the Emergency Department in the majors area.

Your next patient has noticed that they have a facial droop. Please perform a cranial nerve examination. After 6 minutes the examiner will stop you and ask you to summarise back your findings, suggest your differential diagnoses and your initial management plan

Examiner's instructions

The cranial nerve examination should be smooth and respectful towards the patient. Marks are awarded for different parts of the examination as well as the overall impression.

The examination will be followed by questions about a Bell's palsy. You should ask the candidate how to distinguish between an upper and lower motor nerve lesion affecting the facial nerve. You should then tell the candidate that the patient in question shows signs of a lower motor nerve lesion and ask them for a possible cause of this. If they correctly identify Bell's palsy as a cause of a lower motor neurone lesion ask them what is the most common cause of a Bell's Palsy. If they cannot name the syndrome tell them that Bell's palsy is a possible diagnosis. They should know that a herpes virus is often thought to be the cause.

If time allows ask for their steps in the management of a Bell's palsy. They should tell you that the treatment is mainly supportive. Tape to help with eye closure, eye drops etc. Steroids can be useful if started within 72 hours of symptom onset. Acyclovir is sometimes used but its effectiveness has not been reliably documented.

Mark Scheme: Cranial Nerve Examination

Task	Achieved	Not Achieved
Introduces self and washes hands		
Confirms identity and gains consent		
Explains to the patient the nature of the examination		
Asks about sense of smell (I)		
Tests visual fields (II)		
Suggests the use of a Snellen chart and performing ophthalmoscopy. (+/- ishihara chart) (II) Does not need to demonstrate these)		
Correctly assesses eye movements (patient follows a point in a H shape) (III, IV, VI)		
Correctly assesses the pupillary light response and accommodation reflex (III)		
Tests the sensation over the forehead, cheek and mandible (V)		
Tests the muscles of mastication and jaw opening (V)		
Tests the muscles of facial expression (VII)		
Asks about hearing loss and mentions the Weber and Rinne tests as means of further assessment (does not need to demonstrate these) (VIII)		
Mentions but does not perform the gag reflex and testing sensation of the palate (IX)		
Tests motor function of the soft palate: asks patient to say 'aah' and looks for uvula deviation (X)		
Asks patient to turn head and shrug shoulders against resistance (XI)		
Examines tongue movements (XII)		
Thanks patient and carries out the examination in a courteous manner		
Is able to talk through the examination and explain which of the cranial nerves are being tested		
Explains the difference between an upper and lower facial nerve palsy and identifies the syndrome as 'Bell's Palsy'		
Suggests herpes infection as a possible cause of a Bell's palsy and highlights the need for supportive management in Bell's palsy and is aware of steroids +/- acyclovir as possible treatments.		
Examiner's global mark	/5	
Helper's global mark	/5	
Total station mark	/30	

Learning points

- Below is an outline of the cranial nerve (CN) examination. All textbooks and websites will have a slightly different variation on the theme.

- Get used to talking through your examination as you are doing it and explaining which of the cranial nerves you are testing. Make sure you talk to the patient at least at the start and the end to put them at ease.

- Your examination does not have to test each cranial nerve in numerical order. What matters is that you have a system that is logical and makes sense to you. It may help to group the nerves and tests each group in turn. This not only makes your examination look polished but can also help you remember them.

CN	Name	Tests
I	Olfactory	Ask about a change in sense of smell
II	Optic	Test visual fields Suggest using a Snellen chart to test visual acuity Suggest performing ophthalmoscopy Suggest using an ishihara chart for colour vision It would be unlikely that you would need to demonstrate these during a cranial nerve examination station. Mentioning the tests will suffice.
III	Oculomotor	All eye movements apart from those performed by IV and VI Pupillary reflexes: accommodation and light response
IV	Trochlear	Superior Oblique: 'Down and out' eye movement
V	Trigeminal	Test the three sensory branches of the trigminal nerve: Ophthalmic (forehead), Maxillary (cheek) and Mandibular (chin) Test the motor function of the trigeminal nerve: ask the patient to clench their teeth and feel the masseter muscles just superior to the angle of the jaw and temporals muscles over the temples. Test

		the pyerygoids by asking the patient to open their mouth against resistance. Mention the corneal reflex: the patient closes their eye in response to touching the eye with cotton wool. Do not perform this test on the patient as it is uncomfortable.
VI	Abducens	Lateral rectus: abduction of eye
VII	Facial	Motor function of the facial nerve: open eyes as wide as possible and look for symmetrical wrinkling of the forehead. Ask the patient to close their eyes and not to let the examiner open them. Puff out cheeks. Bare teeth. (It's often easier to ask the patient to copy the faces you pull as well as giving them instructions) The facial nerve also supplies taste to the anterior 2/3 of the tongue but this is not routinely tested in the cranial nerve examination
VIII	Vestibulocochlear	Ask about any change in hearing. Crude testing can be performed by rubbing your fingers together next to each of the patient's ears in turn and asking if both sides sound the same. Special tests: Weber's test is a screening test for hearing loss. Place a vibrating tuning fork on the middle of the forehead and ask which side is louder. In a normal examination both sides will sound the same. If the patient hears the sound louder on one side this can mean a conductive hearing deficit in the louder ear or sensorineural hearing loss in the quieter ear. This is easier to establish if the patient can tell you which ear is problematic. Rinne's test finishes the assessment: a vibrating tuning fork is placed on the mastoid process then immediately next to the ear. The patient is asked if the sound is louder in the first or the second position. In a normal ear the sound will be louder in the second position: with the tuning fork next to the ear assessing AIR CONDUCTION which is normally louder. If the sound is louder when the tuning fork is on the mastoid process this suggests that BONE CONDUCTION is louder than AIR CONDUCTION which suggests a conductive hearing loss. Imagine in a conductive hearing deficit that

		there is a pea stuck in the patient's ear. That will result in these findings. It is probably sufficient in most cranial nerve stations to just say that you would use these tests but not actually execute them.
IX	Glossopharyngeal	Sensory innervation of the palate. Suggest but do not execute the gag reflex. Can also test soft touch of the palate. Again, it should be sufficient to mention but not execute this test as it is quite uncomfortable.
X	Vagus	Motor innervation of the soft palate. Ask the patient to say 'aah' and watch for uvula deviation and symmetrical elevation of the palate.
XI	Accessory	Test the sternocleidomastoid muscle by asking the patient to turn their head to look over each shoulder in turn against resistance. Test the trapezius muscle by asking the patient to shrug their shoulders against resistance.
XII	Hypoglossal	Test tongue movements: look at the tongue at rest to look for any fasciculations seen in a LMN lesion. Ask the patient to stick their tongue out and look for deviation. in a LMN lesion the tongue will deviate toward the lesion suggesting muscle weakness on the affected side. In an UMN lesion the tongue will deviate away from the lesion suggesting weakness on the contralateral side.

36. Lower limb neurology

Candidate's Instructions

You are the foundation doctor in the Emergency Department in the minors area.

A 39-year-old gentleman presents to ED after developing severe lower lumbar back pain with associated left sided lower limb numbness and feels he is having difficulties mobilising over the last 5 days. He has had ongoing back issues since having lumbar spinal surgery when he was 25 after a rugby accident.

After 6 minutes the examiner will stop you and ask you to summarise back your findings, suggest your differential diagnoses and your initial management plan

Examiner's Instructions

The candidate is a foundation year doctor in the minors area of ED. A 39-year-old gentleman presents to minors after developing severe lower lumbar back pain with associated left sided lower limb numbness and feels he is having difficulties mobilizing over the last 5 days. He has had ongoing back issues since having lumbar spinal surgery when he was 25 after a rugby accident.

The candidate should assess the lower limbs only in 6 minutes and should examine for:

- Tone
- Power
- Sensation
- Coordination
- Reflexes

The candidate should mention that they would assess for perianal tone and saddle anaesthesia.

With 2 minutes remaining ask the candidate to summarize their findings and to give your their differential diagnoses.

Actor's Instructions

You are a 39-year-old gentleman who presents to ED after developing severe lower lumbar back pain, with associated left sided lower limb numbness and increasing difficulties mobilising over the last 5 days

You have developed weakness in your right leg over the last 5 days after having chronic back pain for approximately 10 years since a rugby accident. However, this 'feels' different.

The back pain originates in the lower back and radiates down into the thigh of your right leg. You have become concerned as you are having difficulties lifting your leg from the hip. You can kick out at the knee as normal and move your foot as normal but your right-sided hip movement is severely restricted and so is eversion of the ankle (the sole of the **foot** increasingly facing away from the other **foot**) .

You also have numbness around your right buttock and feel there is some weakness when you squeeze your bottom cheeks together. Your left leg feels normal. When they check reflexes of the right leg, they are absent at the ankle.

You are concerned that this is a serious spinal injury and that you will need surgery.

Mark Scheme - Lower limb neurology

Task:	Achieved	Not Achieved
Introduces self and washes hands		
Check identity and gains consent		
Explains examination and what it will entail		
Begins by inspection, commenting on wasting, fasciculation's etc		
Assess gait		
Tone bilaterally tested		
Power of the hip		
Power of knee		
Power of ankle		
Power of toes		
Check for clonus		
Sensation: Dermatomal distribution - perform light touch and Mention Pin prick, hot/cold and vibration		
Suggest checking perianal sensation		
Mentions need for PR		
Reflexes - Knees and Ankles		
Coordination (Sliding ankle from knee to foot)		
Checks Babinski plantar reflex		
Checks Proprioception		
Mentions vibration sense		
Methodical approach comparing like for like on left and right side		
Examiner's Global Mark	/5	
Actor / Helper's Global Mark	/5	
Total Station Mark	/30	

Learning Points

- Use the acronym **SWIFT** for remembering what to look for on inspection
    - **S**cars
    - **W**asting of muscles
    - **I**nvoluntary movements – *dystonia / chorea / myoclonus*
    - **F**asciculations – *lower motor neurone lesions*
    - **T**remor – *Parkinson's*

- It is important to revise and learn the myotomes and dermatomes.

- In all patients presenting with back pain the clinician should always consider the possibility of cauda equina. This is an emergency and requires urgent MRI scan of the spine with neurosurgical input.

37. Cerebellar Examination

Candidate's Instructions

You are the foundation doctor in the Emergency Department in the majors area.

You have been asked to perform a cerebellar examination on a 48-year-old male who presents with severe dizziness, sickness, and instability on his feet. You need to ascertain whether this is a cerebellar or labyrinthine disorder as this will affect the management.

After 6 minutes the examiner will stop you and ask you to summarise back your findings, suggest your differential diagnoses and your initial management plan.

Examiner's Instructions

The candidate is a foundation doctor in the Emergency Department in the majors area who has been asked to see a 48-year-old man with unsteadiness and to perform a cerebellar examination and decide upon the likely differential diagnoses and the initial management plan.

Actor's Instructions

You are a 48-year-old male businessman. You were working on the computer when you suddenly became very dizzy and started feeling nauseated and had some vomiting. You find that it is very difficult to walk and you are extremely unsteady on your feet. You needed assistance from your colleagues who took you downstairs and had to help you in and out of their car.

You are normally fit and well and you do not take any regular medications. You had a similar, much less severe episode 3 years ago that lasted for a few hours but resolved spontaneously. You do not have any pain anywhere. You smoke 20 cigarettes a day.

When you are asked to perform heel to shin movements you struggle, and you are unable to walk in a straight line. In fact, when you are standing you find you are swaying quite significantly.

Mark Scheme - Cerebellar Examination

Task	Achieved	Not Achieved
Introduces self and washes hands		
Gains consent and confirms patient identity		
Inspection around bed, patient appearance and posture		
Assesses gait- Stance and balance		
Assesses tandem walking		
Performs Rombergs test		
Assesses for dysarthria		
Checks for nystagmus		
Checks for dysmetric eye movements and poor pursuit		
Assesses / explains one would asses for pronator drift		
Checks for normal arm rebound		
Assess for dysdiadokinesia		
Assesses for past pointing (finger- nose coordination)		
Assesses tone and reflexes in upper limb		
Assesses tone and reflexes in lower limb		
Assesses heel shin coordination		
Thanks patient and summarises positive findings		
Explains would perform cranial nerve and peripheral nerve examination to complete neurological exam		
Suggests head thrust test as further examination for labyrinthine disorders		
Asks for further imaging, such as CT/MRI and referral to Stroke centre		
Examiner's Global Mark	/5	
Actor / Helper's Global Mark	/5	
Total Station Mark	/30	

Learning points

- If caught early, strokes can be treated much more effectively. The presentations of posterior circulation stroke and labyrinthine disorders have some similarities. In cerebellar disease, there can be mild hyporeflexia. In unilateral cerebellar disease, there is deviation to the side of the lesion due to hypotonia.

- In assessment of pronator drift, a slow upward movement of the arm indicates an ipsilateral lesion in the cerebellum. Tandem walking will exaggerate any unsteadiness - It is good at assessing function of the cerebellar vermis – the first to go with alcoholic degeneration. Romberg's test is a test of sensory, not cerebellar ataxia. Slurred staccato speech is typical of cerebellar dysfunction.

- The head thrust test is useful for detecting unilateral vestibulopathy. The patient's head is turned left and right while the patient keeps a fixed gaze on a certain spot. When the head is turned towards the affected side, the vestibular ocular reflex fails and the eyes perform a corrective saccade to refocus on the target. This indicates a positive test for vestibular disease on that side. This is a good test to differentiate between vestibular and brainstem dysfunction.

38. Acute limb ischaemia

Candidate's Instructions

You are the foundation doctor in the Emergency Department in the majors area.

You have been asked to perform an examination of the peripheral vascular system of the lower limbs on a 68-year-old male with an acute onset of left leg weakness and pain 3 hours ago. He has a history of angina and has been recently diagnosed with atrial fibrillation.

After 6 minutes the examiner will stop you and ask you to summarise back your findings, suggest your differential diagnoses and your initial management plan.

Examiner's Instructions

This is an examination of the lower limbs only. If the candidate offers to examine the cardiovascular system, it is not necessary. If the candidate offers to examine the abdominal aorta or do ABPI, this will also not be necessary but mark this down as offered.

At 2 minutes left in the OSCE ask the candidate to stop and summarise their findings, ask for the correct diagnosis and their management plan as well as any other investigations/examinations they would perform. At this stage examination of the abdominal aorta or ABPI can be offered if not done so before.

Actor's instructions

You are a 68-year-old man with a 3 hour history of weakness and pain in your left leg, the candidate will introduce themselves, and you will consent to the examination of your legs. You will decline pain relief or a chaperone if offered.

If the candidate asks you to wiggle your toes or move your legs below your hip, you cannot. You feel pain if the candidate squeezes your left calf on examination.

Mark Scheme - Acute limb ischaemia

Task	Achieved	Not Achieved
Introduces self and washes hands		
Checks identity and gains Consent		
Offers pain relief and chaperone		
Exposes patient legs to the groin		
Inspection of both legs for skin changes and muscle wasting		
Inspects both heels and toe web spaces		
Assesses patient to wiggle toes (gross motor assessment)		
Palpation of both legs for temperature		
Palpation of both legs for pain		
Palpates both femoral pulses		
Palpates both popliteal pulses		
Palpates both Posterior tibial pulses		
Palpates both dorsalis pedis pulses		
Assesses Capillary refill		
Performs Beurgers test		
Offers to examine abdominal aorta		
Offers Ankle brachial pressure index		
Summarises findings		
Correctly states diagnosis		
Describes appropriate management plan		
Examiner's Global Mark	/5	
Actor / Helper's Global Mark	/5	
Total Station Mark	/30	

Learning points

- Remember the 6 P's of acute limb ischaemia, Pale, pulseless, pallor, paraesthesia, paralysis, and perishingly cold.

- If pulses are difficult to palpate consider using a handheld or portable doppler probe.

- Acute limb ischaemia is a time critical emergency and revascularization within 6 hours is required to prevent permanent muscle necrosis or need for amputation. Paraesthesia, paralysis and pain on squeezing muscles are late signs and may indicate impending irreversible damage.

39. Knee Examination

Candidate's Instructions

You are the foundation doctor working in the Emergency Department. A colleague has already taken a history from this patient but is called away so asks you to examine his knee.

He is a 24-year-old man has been brought to the Emergency department with a painful swollen knee sustained after being tackled by another player whilst playing football yesterday - the other's player's boot went into his left knee. Since then he has had pain on the inside of his left knee and is finding it difficult to walk. Today he woke up and his knee was more swollen so he has come to the ED.

Examiner's Instructions

A 24-year-old man has been brought to the Emergency department with a painful swollen knee. He has an MCL sprain

He reports being tackled by another player whilst playing football yesterday - the other player's boot went into his left knee. Since then he has had pain on the inside of his left knee and is finding it difficult to walk. Today he woke up and his knee was more swollen so he has come to the emergency department.

The foundation doctor in the emergency medicine team has been asked to examine the knee to assess what investigations and treatment are required.

On examining the knee, when the candidate specifies the part of the examination they are doing, you can tell them:

Look- the left knee is generally swollen with bruising over the medial area of the left knee. There is no deformity.
Feel- The joint is not red or hot. It is tender to palpation over the medial joint line and origin/insertion of the MCL
Move- On active movement the knee cannot fully straighten. On passive movement, there is full ROM in the knee.
Ligaments: all ligaments are intact but there is pain on ligamentous testing of the MCL
Neurovascular: Sensation in the lower limb dermatomes are normal. Motor power in the left lower limb is normal except for knee flexion, which has reduced power due to pain.

Femoral, popliteal, posterior tibial and dorsalis pedis pulses are present.

Other joints: The left hip and left ankle examination is normal.

Gait- The patient is limping on the left and partially weight bearing.

Actor's Instructions

You are a 24-year-old man who has been brought to the Emergency department with a painful swollen knee. You report being tackled by another player whilst playing football yesterday - the others player's boot went into your left knee. Since then you have had pain on the inside of your left knee and are finding it difficult to walk. Today you woke up and your knee was more swollen so you have come to the emergency department.

You have already spoken to another doctor and given your history. Now the junior doctor in the emergency medicine team has been asked to examine the knee.

When examined, you can tell the candidate:

The knee is more swollen than usual. When they feel your knee, you can tell them it hurts on the inside of your left knee when it is touched.

When they move your knee, you can tell them it's too painful to straighten it and you can't do it. When they then try to move it you find that you can fully straighten your leg. When they test the ligaments of your knee, you can tell them that it hurts the inside of your knee.

When they test the sensation in your leg, you can report normal and full sensation in all areas.

When they test your knee power compared to the right side, it is slightly weaker.

When they test other joints, you find there are no tender areas and you have full range of movement.

On walking you are limping on your left leg due to knee pain.

Mark Scheme: Knee Examination

Task	Achieved	Not-Achieved
Washes hands, introduces self.		
Checks identity and gains consent.		
Starts with inspection from the end of the bed: General appearances of patient - are they unwell?		
Quickly checks hands, mouth and eyes- for any signs of rheumatological disease.		
Inspects the knee from front and side comparing it to the right knee, for swelling, deformity, redness, bruising, symmetry, inflammation.		
Inspects the back of the knee & popliteal fossa		
Palpates the knee- along the joint line, at the back and over the patella, for tenderness.		
Palpates the knee temperature.		
Assess the knee for effusion- patella tap or brush test.		
Asks the patient to actively flex and extend the knee.		
Passively moves the joint.		
Tests the ACL, PCL, MCL and LCL.		
Completes McMurray's manoeuvre (or similar) to test for meniscal injury.		
Tests sensation of left leg in dermatomal regions, comparing to right leg.		
Tests motor power in lower limb myotomes.		
Checks all lower limb pulses.		
Specifies they would examine the joint above and joint below also.		
Assess the gait of the patient.		
Considers all causes of knee pain/swelling during the examination (i.e. septic arthritis, arthropathy)		
Covers the patient after the examination		
Examiner's Global Mark	/5	
Actor / Helper's Global Mark	/5	
Total Station Mark	/30	

Learning points

- Maintaining the basic principles of Look, Feel, Move then Special tests will hold you in good stead in the OSCE but also in the clinical setting. You should also always remember to examine the joint above and joint below, especially in children and the elderly as it can be hard for them to localise where the pain is coming from.

- The medial collateral ligament is found on the inside of the knee and any damage to it is called a sprain. There are different severities of sprain including:

    - First degree sprain: only a few ligament fibers are damaged and the knee will often heal in 3-4 weeks.

    - Second degree sprain: The ligament is still intact but there is more extensive damage to the ligament fibers.

    - Third degree sprain: Complete rupture of the ligament.

- When there is third degree medial collateral ligament sprain, it is very important to also assess the anterior cruciate ligament and menisci also as there is a high likelihood that these are also damaged. Injury of all three is called the 'triad of O'Donoghue', which usually results from a lateral force to the knee while the foot is fixed on the ground.

40. Shoulder Examination

Candidate's Instructions

You are the foundation doctor in the Emergency Department and you are asked to see a 50-year-old woman has self-presented to ED with left shoulder pain after falling from her bicycle onto her left shoulder earlier that day. She is complaining of pain and restricted movements. Please perform a full shoulder examination, you do not need to take a history.

After 6 minutes the examiner will ask you to present your findings and provide the most likely diagnosis.

Examiner's Instructions

The candidate is a foundation doctor in the Emergency Department in the minors area who has been asked to see a 50-year-old woman has self-presented to ED with left shoulder pain after falling from her bicycle onto her left shoulder earlier that day. She is complaining of pain and restricted movements.

The candidate must perform a full shoulder examination but is not required to take a history. After 6 minutes stop the candidate and ask them to summarise back their findings and the likely diagnosis

Actor's Instructions

You are a 50-year-old woman who has self-presented to ED with pain in your left shoulder after falling off of your bicycle, landing onto your left outstretched arm. Since then you have been feeling pain that is worse when you move your arm.

The candidate should first look at both of your shoulders.

They should then palpate both shoulder joints. You should complain of pain as they press on the joint between your collarbone and your shoulder on the left side. You should also indicate to them that you feel that your left shoulder appears swollen and slightly deformed compared to the right side.

The candidate should then ask you to move your arms independently. You should complain of pain when you lift your arm in front of you, particularly once the arm is above shoulder level and when lifting your arm out to the side past your shoulder level.

The candidate will then move your arms themselves, similarly you should complain of pain when they lift your arm in front of you past shoulder level and to the side past shoulder level.

The candidate should perform a test where they hold your left arm across your body, putting pressure on the joint between your collar bone and your left shoulder. Please cry out in pain during this test and complain of a sharp pain between your collar bone and shoulder.

Finally the candidate will test the strength of various muscles around the shoulder. You complain of a sharp twinge in the area between the left collar bone and shoulder during these tests but have good strength.

Mark Scheme: Shoulder Examination

Task	Achieved	Not Achieved
Introduces self, washes hands and checks identity		
Checks identity and gains consent		
Initiates consultation by asking if the patient has any pain and offers analgesia		
Inspects both shoulders for symmetry, swelling and bruising from the front, back and side		
Palpates both shoulders for temperature		
Palpates the sternoclavicular, acromioclavicular and glenohumeral joint lines for tenderness, swelling and crepitus		
Palpates the humerus, humeral head, acromion process, scapula and clavicle bilaterally for bony tenderness		
Palpates the muscle bulk of the deltoid, supra and infraspinatus and trapezius muscles		
Asks patient to perform screening movements (hands behind head and hands behind back)		
Assesses for painful arc		
Assesses active movement of flexion, extension, abduction, internal and external rotation for symmetry, pain and range of movement		
Assesses passive movements as above for range of motion, crepitus, subluxation and pain		
Assesses supraspinatus muscle by testing active abduction against resistance		
Assesses infraspinatus and teres minor muscles by testing active external rotation against resistance		
Assesses subscapularis muscle by testing active internal rotation against resistance		
Tests for acromio-clavicular joint pathology by placing the arm into forced adduction across the chest and palpating the ACJ		
States that they would also examine the C-spine and elbow for a complete evaluation		
States that they would also assess the neurovascular status of the limb		
Summarises examination succinctly		
Correctly identifies diagnosis of acromio-clavicular joint sprain/separation		
Examiner's Global Mark	/5	
Actor / Helper's Global Mark	/5	
Total Station Mark	/30	

Learning Points

- Remembering the basics of most joint examinations will gain you plenty of marks in any joint examination OSCE: correctly expose the joints, always assess and compare both joints, remember to look, feel, move and perform special tests. Finish by stating you would examine the joints above and below as well as the neurovascular status of the limb.

- It is not always possible for exam organisers to provide models with joint pathology, you may have to rely on the patient providing you with cues or you may be examining a normal joint. Do not hesitate to present your findings as those of a normal joint examination if that is the case.

- You do not require an orthopaedic level depth of anatomy knowledge. However, you must know the correct anatomical names of the muscles, joint lines, bones and ligaments that you test in your examination.

41. - PV exam: Removal of lost tampon

Candidate's instructions

You are the foundation doctor in the Emergency Department working in the majors area. You have been asked to see this 23-year-old woman who has presented to the department having lost a tampon.

Please take a focused history, explain and perform a vaginal examination with the equipment provided.

After 6 minutes the examiner will stop you and ask you to summarise back your findings and your initial management.

Examiner's instructions

The candidate has been asked to take a focused history, explain and perform an internal vaginal examination for a patient who has presented with a lost tampon. Please direct the candidate to the model vagina for the practical part of this station.

You will offer to act as a chaperone.

Actor's instructions

You are a 23-year-old woman who has presented to your emergency department with a lost tampon. You are currently in the middle of your period. You placed the tampon in this morning but can no longer feel the strings; you do not think it has fallen out.

You are otherwise fit and well. You have a regular menstrual cycle. You have a long-term partner and use barrier method of contraception. You have not noticed any foul smelling discharge. You do not feel unwell.

You attend the cervical cancer screening programme, you found the smear to be quite uncomfortable and are concerned about what the doctor will have to do to remove the tampon. You feel a bit embarrassed about having to come to see the doctor today.

Mark Scheme - PV exam: Removal of lost tampon

Task	Achieved	Not Achieved
Introduces self to patient, washes hands		
Confirms patient's age and date of birth		
Asks focused history of why patient is here today		
Asks if the patient has any pain, offers analgesia		
Explains that the patient will need a bimanual internal examination		
Explains that the details of the examination		
Obtains verbal consent		
Offers chaperone		
Allows patient to undress in a private manner		
Gets equipment ready, Gloves, speculum, lubricant gel		
Ensures speculum is warm		
Asks patient to get into correct position		
Performs bimanual examination		
Comments on palpating the cervix		
Proceeds to speculum examination		
Inserts speculum on its side and rotates 90 degrees		
Opens speculum and looks for foreign body		
Uses forceps to remove foreign body		
Explains to patient that the procedure is finished, they can get dressed		
Invites any questions		
Examiner's global score	/5	
Patient's Global score	/5	
Total Station Mark	/30	

Learning points

- Obtain consent by explaining the reason for the procedure, the benefits of having it done and the possible complications. Allow time for the patient to clarify any points. Common complications are pain and failure of procedure.

- Always take a sexual and menstrual/pregnancy history in women of childbearing age who present for any reason. All female patients in the ED are pregnant until proven otherwise.

- Patients often feel embarrassed when presenting for intimate examinations, it is useful to acknowledge this and reassure patients that this is a normal part of your job, remain professional at all times.

42. Airway manoeuvres and adjuncts

Candidate's instructions

You are the foundation doctor in the resuscitation room of the ED and have been asked if a final year medical student can shadow you for the day.

The team has received a priority call informing them that a female patient with a reduced GCS is expected to arrive in the department shortly. She is reported to be heavily intoxicated with no evidence of any injuries.

Using the equipment provided explain to the student the basics of airway management. Include in your teaching, basic airway manoeuvres, as well as the selection and insertion of airway adjuncts and devices. You should demonstrate how you would escalate your control of an airway if your initial techniques were unsuccessful.

For the purpose of this station the attachment of oxygen and demonstration of intubation is not required.

Actor's instructions

You are a final year medical student on a placement in the emergency department. You are shadowing a foundation doctor for the day in the resuscitation area. The team gets a priority call informing them that an unconscious female patient is being brought into the emergency department.

You are glad to have the opportunity to watch the foundation doctor manage this patient's airway as you are worried about having to do this once you have qualified and are on the wards. You ask the doctor to talk you through how they will manage the airway of the expected patient. You aren't confident about selecting equipment or your technique with manoeuvres and inserting airway adjuncts and devices. You are also concerned about how to respond if the airway remains compromised despite an intervention.

You have had a practical session in which you have been shown the different airway manoeuvres and pieces of airway equipment but you have never been able to practice this on a mannequin and you have never observed emergency airway management on a real patient. If the foundation doctor offers to demonstrate the equipment you are keen to be shown but you do not need to practice yourself.

Questions to ask if not already covered:

How do you know when you are achieving adequate ventilation?
Are there any situations that a nasopharyngeal airway shouldn't be used?
How can you tell which size of adjunct to use?

Respond well to: enthusiastic, encouraging approach with clear instructions and an opportunity to practice.

Examiner's Instructions

The foundation doctor is working in the resuscitation area of the emergency department. They have been asked to supervise a final year medical student for the day. A priority call is received pre-warning the department of the arrival of an intoxicated female with reduced consciousness. She is likely to require interventions to protect her airway. She has not been involved in a traumatic incident and there is no clinical suspicion of a head injury. The doctor has been asked to demonstrate to the medical student the basic principles of airway management and escalation.

The doctor should demonstrate basic airway manoeuvres, bag valve mask ventilation, the selection and use of airway adjuncts and the use of a supraglottic airway device. They are not expected to demonstrate endotracheal intubation, although they should be aware of this as an advanced method of gaining airway control. They should be aware of the need to urgently seek senior/anaesthetic help when a patient has a compromised airway. They have been asked to focus on the escalation of airway management.

They should establish and address the medical student's learning needs, be supportive and demonstrate an ability to facilitate learning.

Mark Scheme - Airway manoeuvres and adjuncts

Task	Achieved	Not Achieved
Introduces themselves to the student and washes hands		
Establishes student's learning needs		
Establishes existing knowledge and experience		
Sets realistic and achievable learning objectives		
Briefly explains how to assess airway patency and adequate ventilation		
Uses suction to remove any liquid obstruction		
Demonstrates head tilt chin lift correctly		
Demonstrates jaw thrust correctly		
Demonstrates bag valve mask ventilation (one handed or two) correctly		
Explains rationale and demonstrates the use of nasopharyngeal airway		
Demonstrates how to size a nasopharyngeal airway		
Explains rationale and demonstrates the use of oropharyngeal airway		
Demonstrates how to size a oropharyngeal airway		
Explains rationale and demonstrates the use of a supraglottic device		
Explains correctly the process of escalation of airway management if an intervention is inadequate		
Aware of the need to escalate complex cases and the possible need for ET intubation by a senior colleague/ anaesthetist		
Checks the student's understanding		
Gives the student the opportunity to practice		
Encouraging and provides constructive feedback		
Asks if the student has any questions and answers them correctly		
Examiner's Global Mark	/5	
Actor / Helper's Global Mark	/5	
Total Station Mark	/30	

Learning points

- Managing a patient's airway can be complex and frightening and a methodical escalating stepwise approach should be used. it is important to convey to an examiner that you understand that early involvement of senior colleagues/ an anaesthetist is always appropriate if there is potential for airway compromise.

- A sound knowledge of airway manoeuvres, bag valve mask ventilation and basic airway adjuncts and devices is key. Know how they are selected, sized and notable contraindications. Be able to demonstrate how each is inserted.

- Teaching is an integral part of a doctor's job. You need to be able to demonstrate the ability to establish learning objectives, communicate in a clear and appropriate manner and deliver teaching in a supportive and enthusiastic way. Always check the baseline knowledge to avoid over or under pitching your teaching and importantly set realistic and achievable objectives.

43. Oxygen delivery

Candidate's Instructions

You are the foundation doctor in the Emergency Department who has been asked to demonstrate and explain methods of oxygen delivery to a 2nd year nursing student who is starting their placement in the ED.

You will be provided with any equipment required.

Examiner's Instructions

A foundation doctor has been asked to demonstrate and explain methods of oxygen delivery to a nursing student.

Appropriate equipment has been provided. The candidate will be expected to have knowledge of the different types of oxygen delivery methods and how to use them. Knowledge regarding advantages and disadvantages of each method should be sought during the station.

The student nurse has been prompted to pick up pieces of equipment and ask questions if the candidate does not use them.

Actor's Instructions

You are a 2ⁿᵈ year nursing student about to start a placement in an Emergency Department. You are keen to learn more about different ways of administering oxygen to patients.

If asked by the candidate, you are aware that there are different methods to administer oxygen but you have never done so yourself. If the candidates does not use the equipment provided then please prompt them appropriately.

If you are prompted to ask questions by the candidate please ask them about advantages and disadvantages to the different methods.

Mark Scheme: Oxygen Delivery

Task	Achieved	Not Achieved
Introduces self to student, checks identity and washes hands		
Establishes level of previous knowledge of oxygen delivery from student		
Explains purpose of practical session and/or states aims		
Explains that supplemental oxygen may be required in unwell patients		
Appropriately demonstrates how to wear nasal cannulae using mannequin		
Explains maximum flow rates up to 4L/minute delivered by nasal cannulae		
Discusses advantages and disadvantages to using nasal cannulae		
Appropriately demonstrates how to wear face mask using mannequin		
Discusses advantages and disadvantages to using face mask		
Appropriately explains when and why Venturi masks are used		
Understands how various colours of Venturi correspond to different percentages of oxygen delivery		
Appropriately demonstrates how to attach Venturi valve onto face mask		
Explains advantage of controlled oxygen delivery via Venturi		
Appropriately sets up a non-rebreather face mask		
Explains high-flow oxygen via non-rebreather mask is used in medical emergencies		
Asks student to demonstrate a method of oxygen delivery discussed		
Summarises methods of oxygen delivery		
Asks if student has any questions		
Makes suggestions to gain further experience		
Polite and non-judgemental teaching manner throughout		
Examiner's Global Mark	/5	
Actor / Helper's Global Mark	/5	
Total Station Mark	/30	

Learning points

- Oxygen is a drug and as such should be clearly prescribed on a drug chart. This includes documenting flow rate, method of oxygen delivery and target oxygen saturations.

- Controlled oxygen therapy is most accurately delivered by a Venturi mask. The following colours and minimum oxygen flow rates demonstrate percentage oxygen delivery:

  Blue – 24%, 2L/min; White – 28%, 4L/min; Yellow – 35%, 8L/min, Red - 40%, 10L/min, Green – 60%, 15L/min

- In a medical emergency where a patient is unwell or deteriorating, always commence high-flow oxygen (15L via non-rebreather mask). Oxygen therapy can then be titrated subsequently pending results of arterial blood gas sampling. The same is true in patients that are COPD and are at risk of CO_2 retention. The hypoxia will harm the patient before the hypercapnia will so never delay giving high flow oxygen if a patient is unwell.

44. Ear foreign body practical

Candidate's Instructions:

You are the foundation year doctor in the Emergency Department working in the minors area and have been asked to see Tracey a 27-year-old female who has attended the emergency department with "something in her ear" and reduced hearing on that side.

She first noticed this after cleaning her ear with a cotton bud. She is systemically well with normal observations and no other complaints.

Examine Tracey's ear and proceed with the removal of any foreign body you may identify. A selection of instruments has been provided to assist you with the above.

Examiner's Instructions

The candidate is a foundation year doctor in the Emergency Department working in the minors area who has been asked to see Tracey a 27-year-old female who has attended the emergency department with "something in her ear" and reduced hearing on that side.

The patient first noticed this after cleaning her ear with a cotton bud. She is systemically well with normal observations and no other complaints.

Observe the candidate using an auroscope to identify a retained cotton bud tip in the models ear. They should then proceed to remove it with an appropriate instrument.

Actor's Instructions:

The candidate is a foundation year doctor in the Emergency Department working in the minors area. They have been asked to see you, Tracey a 27-year-old female, as you have attended the ED with "something in her ear" and reduced hearing on that side.

You first noticed this after cleaning your ear with a cotton bud. This is something you do every morning so you are unsure why there is suddenly a problem. You are well in yourself with normal observations and no other complaints. You have no medical history of note and don't take any medications.

The candidate should examine the ear and identify a retained cotton bud tip in the models ear. They should then proceed to remove it with an appropriate instrument.

(Ear model to be used in conjunction with patient actor)

Mark Scheme: Auroscopy

Task	Achieved	Not Achieved
Introduces self and washes hands		
Confirms patient name and obtains consent		
Establishes brief history		
Asks permission to undertake the examination and explains procedure		
Positions patient appropriately		
General inspection of ear – erythema, discharge		
Palpates tragus, retracts pinna and palpates mastoid for tenderness		
Examines for pre and post auricular lymphadenopathy		
Checks auroscope function – light working etc		
Attaches appropriate size plastic tip		
Inspects external meatus with auroscope		
Identifies retained cotton bud tip sitting in front of TM		
Selects appropriate instrument for removal – crocodile forceps, plastic tweezers, fine tooth forceps		
Successfully retrieves cotton bud tip		
Inspects tympanic membrane for perforation		
Comments on light reflex, any effusion or erythema, grommets,		
Offers field hearing test/whispered voice hearing test		
Educates patient on the use of cotton buds		
Invites questions		
Thanks the patient		
Examiner's Global Mark	/5	
Actor / Helper's Global Mark	/5	
Total Station Mark	/30	

Learning Points

- Common foreign bodies in the ear that may present to the emergency department include cotton buds, insects, peas, popcorn, beads and chalk. Most foreign bodies are more common in children than adults, which can itself present difficulties with retrieval.

- All efforts should be taken to minimise damage to the external auditory canal and referral to a specialist should be considered instead of repeated attempts to retrieve object.

- Become familiar with wax in all its forms as this often can appear like a foreign body. Take the opportunity to learn what the different presentations of ear pathology looks like.

45. Ophthalmoscopy

Candidate's instructions

You are the foundation doctor in the Emergency Department working in the minors area. A 22-year-old plumber's apprentice Kasia presents to the department with a red painful eye, which started when they were drilling pipes at work without eye protection.

Perform an examination of her eye including ophthalmoscopy.

Examiner's instructions

In this station the candidate should perform an eye examination including ophthalmoscopy on the patient. The history is suggestive of a corneal foreign body or corneal abrasion. They should be able to outline the additional examinations they wish to perform and the expected findings in the context of a corneal abrasion.

The examination should start with inspection of the eye. They should mention everting the eyelids to look for a foreign body but you should tell them that they do not need to do this. They should also examine pupil reactions and extraocular movements. In this context the inspection of the eye is equally or even more important than the ophthalmoscopy and they should not rush straight into using the ophthalmoscope.

You should provide them with a Snellen chart to test visual acuity if they ask for one but it will not be visible in the station. This should form part of their examination. Once they have illustrated that they know how to use the Snellen chart do not let them spend too much time on this. The patient should stand 6 meters away from the chart (provided they are using a 6m chart) and if they normally wear glasses they should have them on. One eye should be examined at a time. The smallest line that can be read represents the visual acuity. If the patient gets 2 or more letters wrong the line above is recorded as their acuity. There will also be text available for close vision and an Ishihara chart for colour vision. They should not spend too much time on this part of the examination either.

They should perform a visual field examination and test pupillary reflexes.

The candidate should talk you through what they are looking for when they are performing ophthalmoscopy.

Once they have finished the examination ask them what other tests they would like to perform. They should tell you that they would like to perform a slit lamp examination with fluorescein dye under a blue light to look for a corneal abrasion. They should be aware that a corneal abrasion would appear as a yellow-green area. They should be aware of how painful a corneal abrasion can be and be aware of the possible need for topical local anaesthetic.

Ask them about management of a corneal abrasion. They should be aware of the need for analgesia, specialist referral and consideration of antibiotics. They should be aware that eye patches are not recommended. They must ask the patient whether or not they wear contact lenses.

Actor's Instructions

The candidate is a foundation year doctor in the Emergency Department working in the minors area. They have been asked to see you, Kasia a 22-year-old female, as you have attended the ED with a red painful eye, which started when you were drilling pipes at work without eye protection.

Ther pain started immediately and you do feel like there is something in your eye. You were given some paracetamol when you first arrived but that hasn't' really helped the pain and you feel the eye is continually watering with your eyelid twitching. Your vision is blurred due to this.

You do not usually wear glasses or contact lens. You are well in yourself with normal observations and no other complaints. You have no medical history of note and don't take any medications.

The candidate should examine your eye fully and suspect a foreign body with likely corneal abrasion and advise further slit lamp examination. They should then proceed to remove it with an appropriate instrument.

(Eye model to be used in conjunction with patient actor)

Mark Scheme: Eye Examination

Task	Achieved	Not Achieved
Introduces self and washes hands		
Checks identity and consents patient		
Explains the nature of the examination to the patient.		
Performs an examination of the eye including ophthalmoscopy in an organised, efficient manner.		
Asks about contact lens use		
Performs a general inspection of both eyes for conjunctival injection or overt pupil asymmetry		
Examines for foreign body with the naked eye		
Explains the need to evert the eyelid to look for foreign body		
Correctly tests visual acuity with a Snellen chart		
Correctly tests visual acuity with small print text		
Correctly tests colour vision with an Ishihara chart		
Tests eye movements		
Tests pupillary reflexes		
Systematically examines the back of the eye		
Thanks patient and carries out the examination in a courteous manner		
Suggests using a slit lamp to complete the examination		
Is aware of the need for fluorescein dye under a blue light to assess for corneal abrasions		
Knows how a corneal abrasion would appear with fluorescein dye under a blue light		
Suggests using local anaesthetic for pain control during the examination		
Is able to discuss further management considerations e.g. specialist referral, consideration of topical antibiotics and current recommendations against the use of an eye patch.		
Examiner's Global Mark	/5	
Actor / Helper's Global Mark	/5	
Total Station Mark	/30	

Learning points:

- It may be tempting in a station like this to reach straight for the equipment, perform the ophthalmoscopy and finish in a few seconds. This examination relies more on external examination than on ophthalmoscopy. Whilst you need to be comfortable using the ophthalmoscope, there are a number of points to be gained before you even pick it up, so make sure you don't miss out on them!

- Corneal abrasions are very painful. This not only distresses the patient, but also significantly limits your examination. So the use of topical anaesthetic agents can be very helpful, as is a lot of reassurance.

- Most places recommend ophthalmology outpatient follow-up after a lesion such as this, to ensure the symptoms are improving, and that a foreign body has not been missed. Rates of bacterial infection after trauma are low but many ophthalmologists recommend antibiotics in the form of topical chloramphenicol.

46. Intraosseous needle insertion

Candidate's Instructions:

You are the foundation year doctor in the Emergency Department in the resus area.

A 60-year-old patient is brought into ED resus with epigastric pain, which is describes as "tearing into my back". The patient is pale, sweaty, clammy and feels very unwell. They also appear to be confused. The heart rate is 150bpm and blood pressure 80/45mmHg. The Ambulance crew state they were unable to gain IV access.

You and your senior have been attempting to cannulate, but have failed. The BP is continuing to fall and his GCS level has dropped. The nurse provides you with an IO needle and drill.

Please explain the indications and demonstrate where and how you would insert an IO needle to gain access.

Examiner's Instructions:

The candidate is a foundation year doctor in the Emergency Department in the resus area who has been asked to see a 60-year-old man who has been brought to ED resus with epigastric pain, which they describe as "tearing into my back". They are pale, sweaty, clammy and feel very unwell. They also appears to be confused. The heart rate is 150bpm and blood pressure 80/45mmHg.

The Ambulance crew state they were unable to gain IV access so the candidate has been asked to place an IO needle.

- Candidate should use IO needle and drill to gain access.

- Candidate should explain the procedure out loud as they perform it

- Candidate should know the indications for IO

- Should explain to the patient what the procedure will entail

- Should perform it using an aseptic technique

Actor's Instructions:

You are a very unwell 60-year-old. who has been brought to ED resus with epigastric pain, which you describe as "tearing into my back". You are pale, sweaty, clammy and feel very unwell. You are confused and slightly delirious, moving around quite a lot.

The paramedic and the doctors have tried to get venous access but have failed multiple times and are now suggesting inserting a metal needle into your bone as a method of giving you drugs and fluids. The have described needing to use a drill which has scared you considerably.

Your heart rate is 150bpm and blood pressure 80/45mmHg and continues to deteriorate so there is no choice but to proceed.

The candidate should explain the indications for the procedure and consent you for it and proceed to place the needle.

Mark Scheme: Intraosseous Needle

Task	Achieved	Not Achieved
Introduces self and washes hands		
Checks patient identity and gains consent		
Explains procedure to patient		
Use of local anaesthetic at insertion point for pain relief (if needed)		
Indication for IO: Failure to gain IV access, Blood sample and IV access is urgently needed and Temporary measure.		
Proximal humerus - Greater tubercle, 1cm above surgical neck		
Proximal tibia - 2 finger breadths below patella, 1-2cm medial to tibial tuberosity		
10ml sterile saline in syringe and prime tubing		
Clean site with chlorhexidine		
Connect needle to drill		
Needle should be perpendicular to bone surface		
Apply gentle pressure until you feel a "give" which is the medullary space		
Stabilise and remove drill from needle		
Remove stylet by turning anti-clockwise		
Dispose of sharps in sharps bin		
Secure with dressing		
Aspirate for bone marrow sample		
Indication for IO removal: extravasation or infection or time period over 24 hours		
Method of removal - Attach a 10ml syringe to the catheter hub, rotate clockwise and pull. Dispose in sharps bin and apply dressing		
Complications → Osteomyelitis, Fracture, Extravasation, Compartment syndrome, Failure		
Examiner's Global Mark	/5	
Actor / Helper's Global Mark	/5	
Total Station Mark	/30	

Learning Points

- Practice makes perfect! Even without the kit, practice the procedure, talking it through yourself so it becomes second nature to you. If you get the chance, in a real life setting to insert an IO, this will consolidate learning

- The IO needle length to be chosen largely depends on the amount of overlying tissue:

    - 45mm (humerus insertion or excessive tissue) yellow
    - 25mm (> 40kg) blue
    - 15mm (3-39kg) red

- Procedural skills in exams are sometimes more about the set up than the procedure itself. Learn how to assemble the IO gun and how to measure out needles and also be aware of your landmarks. These will be important marks in your exam.

47. Urinary Catheter

Candidate's Instructions

You are the foundation year doctor in the Emergency Department working in the majors area and the nurse asks you to see a 67-year-old man with significant abdominal pain who has not passed urine for 12 hours.

Perform a quick history and examination, and explain your next steps in the management. The patient will need a catheter so you will have to prepare for this and insert one using the provided model.

Examiner's Instructions

The candidate is a foundation doctor in the Emergency Department in the majors area who has been see a 67-year-old man with significant abdominal pain who has not passed urine for 12 hours.

They will take a brief history and examination then insert a catheter. After they have inserted the catheter ask which investigations they would like to request and what steps they would take if the procedure had failed.

Actor's Instructions

You are a 67-year-old retired carpenter who has had trouble passing urine for about 6 months. You note that it has been very difficult to have a good stream when passing water, and you can never get a feeling of an empty bladder. You wake up a few times a night to pass water but it often takes a while to start.

You saw your GP about the symptoms a few weeks ago and you had a PSA test but you don't know the result. In the last few days you have been under the weather and have had some burning when passing water. You haven't been able to pass water at all today.

You have mild blood pressure and diet controlled diabetes. You are not currently on any medications. You are widowed and live alone but are feeling quite low mainly die to the worsening sleep you are getting due to waking in the night to pass urine.

The candidate will take a brief history from you, examine you and then recognise the need to insert a urinary catheter. They should explain the process to you, consent you and talk you through it as it happens.

Mark Scheme: Urinary Catheter

Task	Achieved	Not Achieved
Introduces self and washes hands		
Check Identity and gains consent		
Takes history of presenting complaint and urological history		
Examines patient's abdomen		
Requests external genitalia and PR examination		
Asks for bladder scanner		
Explains the need for catheterisation to the patient and takes consent		
Washes hands and uses sterile technique (throughout)		
Prepares trolley with necessary equipment. Uses gloves and gown		
Exposes patient and drapes field around penis		
Retracts foreskin and cleans glans away from urethral meatus		
Changes gloves		
Applies anaesthetic gel and waits appropriate time		
Passes catheter fully and inflates balloon via syringe, asking about pain when inflating		
Pulls catheter until resistance is felt		
Attaches to reservoir bag		
Replaces foreskin over glans		
Thanks patient and recovers them		
Explains would document procedure and residual		
Asks for appropriate Investigations (blood tests, Urine dip)		
Examiner's Global Mark	/5	
Actor / Helper's Global Mark	/5	
Total Station Mark	/30	

Learning points

- When seeing patients with urinary retention, it is important to elicit the urinary symptoms as they will guide us in a differential diagnosis. Hesitancy, poor stream, and feeling of incomplete emptying is normally due to prostatic hyperplasia or prostate cancer. A PR exam is important to determine whether the prostate is Smooth or craggy. We can also check for anal tone during the PR as a cauda equina syndrome can present with urinary symptoms.

- Replacing the foreskin is a must after urethral catheterisation as failure to do so may cause a paraphimosis. This is when the glans swells up and the foreskin cannot be replaced.

- Check a urine dip and the renal profile (electrolytes, urea, and creatinine) after inserting a catheter. Patients can go into diuresis due to increased urea and salt retention, which needs to be lost. There is also as a reduced concentration gradient in the loop of Henle (due to low flow), which does not recover immediately after the obstruction is relieved. Sometimes patients in retention need IV fluids to aid subsequent losses.

48. ABG interpretation

Candidate's Instructions

You are the foundation year doctor in the Emergency Department working in the resus area.

You have just assessed John, a 66-year-old man with 2 days history of worsening shortness of breath on a background history of COPD who has been brought in by ambulance. He is breathing oxygen at 15L per minute via non re-breathe bag.

Please analyse the following arterial blood gas and explain your findings to a medical student who is shadowing you today.

ABG
Name: John
Date of birth: 10/04/1950
Date: 15/09/2016, Time 10:26 am

$$PH - \quad 7.150$$
$$PO_2 - \quad 12.9$$
$$PCO_2 - \quad 9.7$$
$$HCO_3 - \quad 39$$
Base excess : +10.5

Actor's Instructions

You are a 3ʳᵈ year medical student attached to ED resus. A doctor has just received the results of an arterial blood gas. You will ask the doctor to explain the results to you.

You have read about ABG's and have seen one normal ABG before, but a doctor has never explained how to interpret and act on an abnormal ABG before.

Throughout the teaching session you would like the following questions answered if not done so by the candidate:

- How will the doctor act on the ABG findings or what will their management plan be?

- What is base excess?

- Is there much other information a typical ABG analysis/readout can give?

Examiner's Instructions

The candidate is a foundation year doctor in the Emergency Department working in the resus area. They have a medical student shadowing them today who is keen to be taught about data interpretation.

They have just assessed John, a 66-year-old man with 2 days history of worsening shortness of breath on a background history of COPD who has been brought in by ambulance. He is breathing oxygen at 15L per minute via non re-breathe bag.

They have performed an arterial blood gas and should now explain the findings to the medical student in a structured and succinct manner.

Appropriate management plan includes, but not limited to; blood tests, chest x-ray, trial of oxygen therapy to keep Sats 88-92 %, or NIV/BiPAP and critical care referral, nebulisers/steroids and repeat ABG after intervention.

Starting NIV prior to obtaining a chest x-ray is not an appropriate management plan.

The examiner's role is to observe only and not to ask any direct questions.

Mark Scheme: ABG Interpretation

Task	Achieved	Not-Achieved
Introduces self and washes hands		
Establish student's current level of knowledge/understanding		
Sets specific objectives of this learning session		
Systematic approach to analysing ABG		
Brief overview of history/describes clinical context		
Confirms patient details from which ABG was taken		
Confirms time ABG was taken		
States oxygen rate delivered		
Determines PH status Acidotic/alkalosis		
Comments on level of hypoxia		
Explains respiratory component		
Explains metabolic component		
Explains base excess correctly		
Establishes primary disturbance (respiratory acidosis)		
Establishes compensation (metabolic)		
Gives overall diagnosis (Type 2 respiratory failure)		
Describes appropriate management plan		
Has some knowledge of other components displayed on typical ABG		
Summarises learning points		
Asks if student has any further questions		
Examiner's Global Mark	/5	
Actor / Helper's Global Mark	/5	
Total Station Mark	/30	

Learning points

- Remember to compare the pO2 to rate of oxygen being delivered to determine level of hypoxia. As a rough rule of thumb the pO2 should be comparable to the percentage oxygen delivered minus 10 eg 15L via non re -breathe bag at a FiO2 percentage of 85% should manifest an approximate pO2 in the blood of 85-10 =75

- Always do a Chest X-ray prior to starting NIV. One of the causes of COPD exacerbation can be a pneumothorax that will be made worse with NIV.

- When teaching junior colleagues remember to establish their current level of knowledge/skill. State learning objectives prior to the session, summarise the points after and ask for any questions. Giving them resources such as websites or podcasts to go away and access is a good way to consolidate learning.

49. ECG Interpretation

Candidate's Instructions:

You are the foundation year doctor in the Emergency Department working in the resus area.

A third year medical student doing their placement in the emergency department has come to you asking how to interpret an ECG. They need to present the ECG in the correct manner to their clinical supervisor later and will be marked on their presentation, interpretation, explanation and recognition of patterns of ischaemia on ECGs.

This is the ECG they show you:

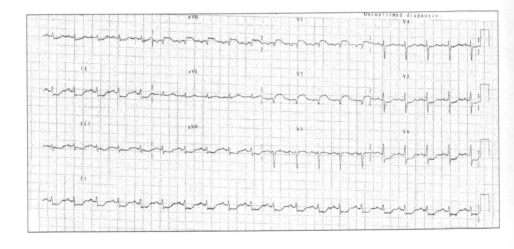

Examiner's Instructions:

The candidate is a foundation doctor in the Emergency Department in the majors area.

A medical school student doing their placement in the ED has approached the foundation doctor in emergency medicine asking them how to interpret an ECG (below).

This is the student's first clinical placement during medical school and they state they are unsure how to interpret and present the ECG to their clinical supervisor. The student explains they will be marked on their presentation and interpretation of the ECG and also their explanation to how to recognise patterns of ischaemia on ECG.

You are there to assess how the candidate explains ECG interpretation in the context of this ECG showing anterior ischaemia.

Actor's Instructions:

You are a third year medical student who is doing their first clinical placement in a hospital in the emergency department. As part of your medical school portfolio, your supervising consultant has asked you to interpret an ECG (seen below) and also be able to explain how to recognise patterns of ischaemia on ECG.

You are worried about getting a good mark so find the foundation doctor In emergency medicine and ask for their help in explaining interpretation of ECGs using the one below as an example as well as asking them to explain how to recognise patterns of ischaemia.

When asked, you tell them you have seen ECGs in lectures but never interpreted or presented one yourself. You say you know there is a system to it but you can't quite remember it and found it previously difficult to understand.

At each stage of the explanation, you ask how this is interpreted in the context of the ECG.

Mark Scheme : ECG

Task	Achieved	Not-Achieved
Introduces self and builds rapport		
Ascertains exactly what their aims and objectives are of the session.		
Clarifies what clinical level they are at and what they know already.		
States the student must first confirm the patient's name, age, ECG date/time and presenting complaint.		
Explains the need to check paper speed first (25mm/sec) and how to calculate the ECG rate (300/R-R)		
Explains how to assess rhythm		
Explains a method for estimating ECG axis.		
Explains how to look for p waves and form of the p wave.		
Shows how to calculate PR interval		
Shows how to calculate QRS duration		
Explains to the student to look for pathological Q waves and their significance.		
Briefly explains QT interval.		
Explains about changes seen in ST segment in STEMI and NSTEMI		
Explains about changes seen in T wave in STEMI and NSTEMI		
Explains how ischaemic changes in different leads show a pattern of ischaemia in a particular part of the heart (inferior, lateral and anterior ischaemia)		
Summarises the teaching session succinctly.		
Asks if the student has any further questions.		
Refers to and uses the ECG to refer to each part of the teaching points.		
Speaks in language and context appropriate to the level of the student.		
Gives a clear explanation of ECG interpretation whilst maintaining good rapport with the student.		
Examiner's Global Mark	/5	
Actor / Helper's Global Mark	/5	
Total Station Mark	/30	

Learning points

- Anterior STEMI is due to the occlusion of the LAD. It is usually seen as ST elevation with Q wave formation in leads V1-V6 and the high lateral leads (I and aVF). Reciprocal ST depression may be seen in the inferior leads (III and aVF).

  The precordial leads can be classified as: Septal (V1-V2), Anterior (V3-V4) and Lateral (V5-V6).

- Inferior STEMI can be seen in ECG's as ST elevation in lead II, III and aVF, development of Q waves in these leads also and reciprocal ST depression in aVL.

- ECG changes seen in posterior infarct include Tall broad R waves and upright T waves in V1-V3, a dominant R wave in V2 (bigger than the S wave) and also horizontal (as opposed to sloping) ST depression in V1-V3. There may also be some reciprocal ST depression in aVR.

50. CXR interpretation

Candidate's Instructions

You are the foundation year doctor in the Emergency Department working in the majors area. You have reviewed an 18-year-old who presented with sudden onset shortness of breath and right sided chest pain. After taking a history and examining him you sent him for a CXR.

The ED nurse has informed you that the CXR images are available. She asks for your help interpreting the x-ray.

You will have an image of a chest x-ray. You are required to interpret the CXR and explain your methods and conclusions to the nurse as you go along.

Examiner's Instructions

The candidate is a foundation doctor in the Emergency Department in the majors area.

They have seen a 18-year-old man who presented with sudden onset shortness of breath and right-sided chest pain has been seen in the ED. After taking a history and being examined he was sent for a CXR. The ED nurse has called to report that the CXR images are available. She asks for help interpreting the x-ray.

An image of a chest x-ray is provided to the candidate. The candidate is asked to interpret the CXR and explain their methods and conclusions to the nurse.

Actor's Instructions

The candidate is a foundation doctor in the Emergency Department in the majors area.

They have seen a 18-year-old man who presented with sudden onset shortness of breath and right-sided chest pain has been seen in the ED. After taking a history and being examined he was sent for a CXR.
You are the ED nurse in the Majors area and have asked the doctor to explain the CXR findings to you. You will be attending a course on CXR interpretation for nurses soon and would like to get a head start.

The candidate should then proceed to take you through a systematic approach to interpreting the chest x-ray using the chest x-ray available and commenting on any abnormalities he identifies.

When the candidate identifies an abnormality and makes a diagnosis (pneumothorax), you ask what a pneumothorax is. You should mention the pneumothorax only if the candidate has mentioned it first.

You then ask the candidate how he could tell this was a pneumothorax from the x-ray, unless he has already spontaneously done so.

Mark Scheme: CXR Interpretation

Task	Achieved	Not Achieved
Introduces self to nurse		
Confirms correct patient details and date on the x-ray		
Demonstrates a structure approach to chest x-ray interpretation		
Explains how to differentiate between an AP and PA film		
Explains how to assess film adequacy including exposure, inspiration and if whole chest included		
Mentions the importance of recognizing a rotated film		
Comments on trachea and airway patency, looking for deviation, masses and foreign bodies		
Explains clearly that all bones should be assessed for abnormalities- ribs, clavicle, scapula and humerus		
Comments on the importance of assessing the breasts and other soft tissues		
Explains how to assess the heart size, contours and retro-cardiac space on x-ray		
Describes the normal mediastinum appearance on x-ray		
Explains the importance of examining the diaphragm outline on x-ray and the significance of the costo-phrenic angle		
Mentions the need to assess the hilar shadows		
Mentions the need to examine any part of the abdomen seen on the x-ray for obvious abnormalities		
Demonstrates the landmarks used to recognize each lobes on x-ray		
Describes the abnormalities seen in the lung field of the x-ray		
Correctly identifies the abnormality as a pneumothorax		
Correctly explains to the nurse what a pneumothorax is		
Correctly explains to the nurse why this appearance of suggestive of a pneumothorax		
Stresses the importance of also commenting on any obvious lines, leads and tubes		
Examiner's Global Mark	/5	
Actor / Helper's Global Mark	/5	
Total Station Mark	/30	

Learning Points

- Data interpretation OSCEs are used to demonstrate that you will be able to recognize key clinical situations. However, the benefit of using an OSCE as opposed to a written question is to assess whether you have a clear understanding of the tests and a systematic approach to interpreting results.

- It is also an excellent way to test your communication and teaching skills. You will find yourself teaching informally on a nearly daily basis once you are qualified. Remember that you are talking to a qualified colleague, not a layperson.

- Although not asked specifically in this OSCE, remember that when you are asked to comment on a set of blood results or imaging, you should always check on the clinical status of the patient first and then comment on any obvious abnormality first. Then, proceed to using a systematic approach to summarize the findings and conclude with your overall impression.

References

Lim et al. BTS guidelines for the management of community acquired pneumonia in adults:update 2009. A quick reference guide. Thorax 2009.

Alvarado, A (May 1986). "A practical score for the early diagnosis of acute appendicitis.". Annals of Emergency Medicine. 15 (5): 557–64. doi:10.1016/S0196-0644(86)80993-3

Ohle et al.: The Alvarado score for predicting acute appendicitis: a systematic review. BMC Medicine 2011 9:139

For the full ALS algorithm see www.resus.org.uk

Joint British Diabetes Societies Inpatient Care Group. The Management of Diabetic Ketoacidosis in Adults. March 2010

Printed in Great Britain
by Amazon